WHY NOT LIVE A LITTLE LONGER?

Herbert Ellis, MD

MINERVA PRESS
LONDON
MONTREUX   LOS ANGELES   SYDNEY

WHY NOT LIVE A LITTLE LONGER?
Copyright © Herbert Ellis MD 1997

ISBN 1 86106 658 9

First Published 1997 by
MINERVA PRESS
195 Knightsbridge
London SW7 1RE

Printed in Great Britain for Minerva Press

WHY NOT LIVE A LITTLE LONGER?

For Nat Armstrong
in appreciation of his wise indoctrination of the author into
the mysteries of medicine, whilst serving as his House
Physician in 1944.

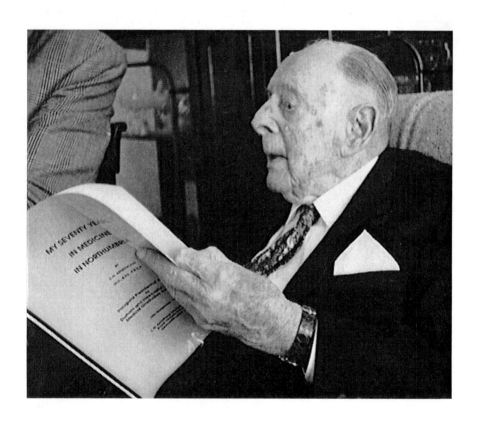

Dr C. N. Armstrong shortly after celebrating his 100th birthday.

Acknowledgement

For permission to quote selected material, thanks to:
Oxford University Press – *Oxford Textbook of Sports Medicine*.
Little Brown – *Origins Reconsidered* by Richard Leakey and Roger Lewin (1992).
Jon Nicholl, medical statistician at the Medical Care Research Unit, Sheffield University (personal communications).
My gratitude also goes to Robert Kruszynski, Department of Palaeoanthropology, Natural History Museum, London, for helping to identify the origins of human speech.
My thanks to Tony Ferguson, himself a former pupil of Dr Armstrong, Glen Byrom and Duncan Lovell for producing photographic confirmation that it *is* possible to 'live a little longer'.
To my many friends, who actively encouraged the completion of this work – sometimes, I suspect, with self-interest at heart! In particular, my thanks go to Admiral Ian Robertson; to Dr Tony Blowers for reading the text; and to Professor Brian Livesley for imparting his vast experience of terminal caring.
A special thanks to the Right Reverend Michael Mann, KCVO, for writing a foreword, and so filling a gap on the subject of faith.
And to my friend and agent, Gerald Pollinger, for his tireless efforts to correct my grammar!
Finally, for my personal well-being, to my wife, Jean (who looks only slightly older now!). Thank you, my dear, for your tolerance, encouragement and patience while *Why Not Live A Little Longer?* evolved.

By the same author:

Hippocrates RN

Published by Minerva Press, 1997.

About the Author

Herbert Ellis was born in Newcastle-upon-Tyne and was educated at Oundle School. He qualified in medicine, at Durham University, in 1944 and joined the Royal Navy's medical branch, at the same time developing a deep and lasting interest in human factors (ergonomics), which influenced the course of his life.

Dr Ellis had been introduced to aviation at the age of two by his father, a Royal Flying Corps pilot in the First World War and subsequently a co-founder of the Newcastle Aero Club. He seized an opportunity to learn to fly in the Fleet Air Arm, before being sent to Farnborough. There he indulged himself by flying anything on offer, including many varied and unusual types of aircraft being developed at that time. He always wore his father's RFC wings under the lapel of his uniform and in later years was to teach his son, Christopher, to fly. His grandson, James Deakin, is a fixed wing pilot, thus making four generations of aviators.

Dr Ellis was instrumental in furthering many developments in human aspects of aircraft operation, both in Britain and America, where he served for a time with the United States Navy. He participated in research into the field of accelerations and their effects on the human body in space. These experiments left Dr Ellis with some personal structural damage, and are related in his autobiography, *Hippocrates RN*.

Constrained by financial problems, he retired from the Royal Navy in 1959 in the rank of Surgeon Commander. He spent ten years in commerce, achieving financial success, but at the cost of his marriage. This resulted in considerable disillusionment about human nature, especially when it becomes poisoned by money. (See the chapter on 'Argentosis'.)

After a ten-year absence from it, Dr Ellis was struck with how medicine had changed, not so much in terms of treatments themselves, but in the application of treatment, together with the doctor-patient relationship. Partly from self-interest, he began to address the twin subjects of human frailty and gerontology, thus providing the subject matter for considerable parts of this book.

Before retiring, he served for twelve years in St John Ambulance, rising to the highest position as Chief Commander for three years and leaving his mark on the organisation in the process.

Inherently shy, he came to realise that elderly people are most appreciative of considerate attention, the administration of which, in turn, served to boost his own self-confidence. Now, in his 'retirement' in Sussex, he is sustained by his wife Jean.

Foreword

Herbert Ellis has had a distinguished and varied medical career, giving him wide experience in many aspects of health and the workings of the human body. He now uses this experience to pose a number of questions about life in general, and death in particular. Death is an event which every one of us will have to face sooner or later; it has become almost a 'forbidden subject'.

Although we spend a great deal of time looking into the future, and in trying to anticipate events, many of us seem to be extremely shy and reluctant to contemplate our own ends. And yet death is universal, it affects all of us whether we be prince or pauper; secondly, it is inevitable, for none of us can avoid passing through that final mysterious doorway; and thirdly, death carries with it a sense of finality tinged with the tragic.

Throughout this book, Dr Ellis emphasises, rightly in my view, the importance of our quality of life. There is a sense, perhaps, in which we have placed too much emphasis upon the length of life, and not enough upon the quality of those years which we are vouchsafed. There are many aspects to the quality of life which each of us is able to enjoy, and their value will depend upon the personal character of the individual. For instance, when my son was killed at the age of twenty-four years, a close friend wrote that his life had been 'like a shooting star'; how does one make a value measurement of twenty-four years lived to the full, in comparison to another life, say, of eighty years, equally full, but of grief and pain? For quality has a dimension that goes beyond mere length of years, and which involves the ability to live each day to the uttermost.

Another way of measuring quality must involve the enjoyment of good health, and the absence of pain. Someone who is dying of a very painful inoperable form of cancer may feel that their quality of life has diminished to such an extent that they no longer wish to be kept alive by medical skill. And yet a young airman in the RAF who lost both his eyes and both his hands in an explosion, has overcome all his disabilities with such courage and humour that no one could say that the quality of his life has been anything but inspiring.

Yet another aspect could involve a deep sense of fulfilment and contentment; there are people who decline advancement in their chosen career when it means moving from the area in which they live, either because of family or educational ties, or because they believe that the area offers a better quality of life than would a move to a less attractive area. Others may find fulfilment in the work which they do and in their ability to contribute, no matter where that contribution is made.

Dr Ellis draws attention to another question which needs to be answered when we think about what makes up the quality of life. A balance has to be struck between material and spiritual values. Too often this balance is lost when too much emphasis is placed upon one side. Our contemporary world does tend to emphasise the material aspects of our lives, but this tendency in itself provokes a reaction in the opposite direction. A lack of balance seldom contributes to an optimum solution.

Those who hold a religious faith are frequently chided for being 'out of date' and 'irrelevant', whilst suggestions are made for ways in which they might become more relevant. The difficulty which such people face in accepting such well-meant suggestions lies in the balance which they believe should be struck between the material and spiritual aspects of the human psyche. There is no such thing as a value-free judgement, and too often the judgements that we do make are loaded either to one side or the other. Those who espouse material values can be irritated by the apparent naivety and elusive nature of so-called spiritual values, whilst those interested in the spiritual will be chary of relaxing what they feel to be high standards and ideals in the hope that a lowering of standards, as they see it, may bring material rewards.

It is understandable that material values should seem to predominate, for the material is concerned with rational, quantifiable facts which can be substantiated by proof. The spiritual side of man is concerned with the intuitive and with feelings. We sometimes forget that the intuitive is just as real as the material, but to the rational mind the difficulty is that it is not subject to logic and reason, only to experience. The paradox is that the material seldom offers an end in itself, giving only transient satisfaction; its real rewards lie in its ability to be the means to the end of attaining a sense of achievement and the fulfilment of the human spirit.

It is also worth remembering that the enormous advances in our knowledge through science and technology are now producing problems which are essentially moral in nature. Let us take, for instance, just one example: the advances in medical practice which have been so spectacular, and with which this book is so concerned. Many of the treatments achieved through this increase in skill and knowledge are extremely expensive to perform. Given the scarcity of resources, and especially financial resources, doctors are increasingly faced with the dilemma of who should benefit, and who should fail to benefit. The concept of a National Health Service which is available to all seems to slip further and further out of our reach. Then how should the choice be made as to who should benefit, and who should be left to suffer, or even to die? Society is placing a huge burden on to the shoulders of medical men in asking them to take such moral decisions.

Herbert Ellis has performed a valuable service in writing this provocative (in the best sense of the word) and challenging book. As with a good sermon, not everyone will agree with all the suggestions the author makes, but the questions need to be put, and the answers pondered upon by all of us.

Rt. Rev. M.A. Mann, KCVO

Preface

When I was cajoled into putting together some thoughts and facts on the subject of death, I was first alarmed, then uneasy at having to face the topic, for hitherto, one often humdrum day seemed to follow another, each one taken for granted, and I never questioned why this routine should not continue indefinitely.

As an ephemeral subject, death can be joked about and kept at bay. One may remains detached, as long as related topics (wills, obituaries) do not precipitate strong feelings. The reality of death is different, and to emphasise the complacency with which the subject is regarded, it was impressed upon me that the word 'death' should not feature in the title of my work ('puts people off, old boy'). In the manner of one applying a tranquilising balm, an adviser finally instructed me that 'you'd better make it light-hearted – like your other literary effort.'[1]

Reflecting on this advice, I realised that we do tend to avoid the subject as a serious topic of conversation, with the possible exception of nervous attempts to make fun of death (take, for example, the phrase 'living death', which implies that death may not really herald the end of life). My task thus fell to reconciling the two anachronistic images of death. Death, though inevitable, is not necessarily imminent, and thus it is easy to focus on life.

But before leaving the subject of death, consider the manner in which it is shunned in other ways, such as through the failure to grant the Royal Warrant. One never sees a hearse inscribed 'by Royal appointment to HRH...' and I have yet to see an undertaker feature in the birthday honours list ('OBE for services to the dead'). Nor do I recall reading an appropriate obituary of a funeral director to lighten the daily lavishly worded appreciations of persons from every other walk of life – the diplomatic service, the armed forces,

---

[1] Herbert Ellis, *Hippocrates RN*, published by Minerva Press.

the Church (as near as obituaries get to undertakers), and many others. But not even a gravedigger gets a mention ('MBE for being unable to do for himself what he had done selflessly for so many others'). With the revitalisation of the honours system perhaps this might be rectified.

In proceeding to investigate the subject matter, and in studying it dispassionately, 'death' turned out to be, paradoxically, a most lively subject, and the deeper it was examined, the more one's attention was directed back to life itself, reinforcing the impulse to continue living. Hence the title of this book.

To conclude this brief preface I can only pass on my own conclusion: that I find, in my seventy-seventh year of life, that the eighth decade of living is proving to be the best one of all – brimming over with liveliness, fun and enjoyable living.

May you find the same.

Contents

"You are old, Father William," the young man said
"And your hair has become very white;
And yet you incessantly stand on your head –
Do you think at your age it is right?"

"In my youth," Father William replied to his son,
I feared it might injure the brain;
But now I'm perfectly sure I have none,
Why, I do it again and again."

From *Alice In Wonderland* by Lewis Carroll (1832–1885)

Chapter One
Introduction

Much of this story may well seem familiar and stir memories, some pleasant, others less so, but that is the patchwork of all our lives. If it stimulates introspection, and if, as a result, some lives are enriched, as mine has been, then it will have been worthwhile putting these thoughts together. For myself, I look back to the many and varied people I have met and often befriended, from every walk and stratum of life. I have learned much from their philosophy and experience, as their stories unfolded.

They have renewed my faith in the human race in the knowledge that, notwithstanding the widespread disenchantment with human attitudes that so widely abounds today, there are many good people around to converse with and with whom one can exchange pleasantries. To find that these same people can rise to crises in their lives, which make my own seem like a Sunday-school outing, makes me feel humble indeed.

I have coined two philosophies from my experiences, which have stood me in good stead in difficult times:

Life isn't fair

and

The best time to approach traffic lights is when they are at red... the position can only get better.

Adopt these two philosophies and you won't be disappointed! With advancing years, the corollary of this is that whenever one is asked, 'How are you?', my stock reply now is, 'Well, I woke up this morning; didn't need helping out of bed (which was not wet or soiled), didn't need help to bathe, to dress – now *that's* living!'

The Task

When, eventually, I was persuaded to commence writing this book, one early decision had to be made:

Was the objective to be how to extend and maximise the quality of life, both in the medium and long term? Or, was it to extend life for as long as possible, irrespective of its quality, also in the medium and long term?

In the event, and in many ways, both objectives have been covered. As to which appeals, the choice must be yours!

> *The failure is not the man who was called before he was ready, but rather the man who was ready... but never called.*

Anon

So, though it was tempting to wait and just see what lay around the next corner, time was running out, so here it is – warts and all. But then... life is just like that!

It has taken over three years to collate the material for this book. The subject matter seemed endless so eventually a decision had to be made to put it all down, albeit incomplete, and get it into print, still leaving many areas uncovered and questions unanswered.

Whilst collecting material I was impressed by the frequency with which the subject of death arose in the course of a day, beginning with the perusal of the obituaries in the paper, with friends developing threatening or actual serious illnesses, with deaths (some unexpected and sudden), near deaths on the roads, painful deaths, reading about '...died peacefully, after a long fight...', even jokes about death. The one common factor was the finality of it all when it happened, and that it could not be avoided. A considerable number of persons, professions, and tradesmen become involved following the moment of death ('act' of death somehow seems incongruous), and we shall be looking at some of these 'callings' later. The medical profession, unless jurisprudence is involved, takes leave of absence quite soon, leaving the others to 'tidy up'.

The clergy must be presumed to have a particular sensitivity regarding the subject of death for they have a significant role to play, a role which is primarily supportive, though stops short of participation, not dissimilar to the 'despatcher' who blows a whistle, then waves a stick to send a train off. Indeed, musing about this, I once gave a bishop a whistle from a Christmas cracker suggesting that it might help him in his duties, but he didn't share my sense of humour!

The supportive, but not participative role of the clergy would explain why the vicar in the following anecdote displayed clear symptoms of paranoia!

A vicar was having his breakfast and reading the morning paper. His wife, who was sitting at the other end of the breakfast table, heard the paper rustling, and, although she couldn't see her husband's face she realised that it was shaking and became concerned for her husband's well-being. She asked him if he was all right, to which he replied,

"No. I'm reading my own obituary and it's just not good enough. I am very upset."

His wife realised that she would not be able to console him and suggested that he should phone the bishop and seek guidance. The vicar agreed, called the bishop and said,

"My Lord Bishop, Cuthbert here, sorry to bother you but I have just been reading my own obituary in this morning's newspaper and it is just not good enough."

There was a long pause, and then the bishop replied, "Oh dear, but first, er... tell me... where are you speaking from?"

A difficulty arose at an early stage of my researches, namely the question of how to conform to the accepted literary form of having a beginning, a middle and an end. Eventually, from deference to the subject, it seemed not unreasonable to start with 'the end'.

It also seemed logical to regard the act of dying only as the end product of living, and, unless a person's life had been productive, enjoyable and happy, then the final act of death could only be a disappointment, for what else could a service of remembrance to celebrate the life of so-and-so be, without happy and joyous memories? In this sense, death might be regarded as a victory, which seems a much more positive approach to the whole subject.

I have enjoyed one significant advantage in that, from a professional medical standpoint, I was able to draw upon the experiences of over ten thousand ordinary people, and in so doing have been able to establish a subjective interpretation of objective findings. In the following work, I intend to examine:

1) *Stress.* Stress and stress-related factors afflict all of us in varying degrees throughout the course of life with some effect on health. Occasionally, one might have been inclined to answer the question in the title with, 'Why indeed live any longer?'

And I shall include:

2) Brief descriptions, with illustrative case histories, of some of the commoner afflictions which are likely to affect many of us, and the commoner life-threatening conditions, as well as those likely to erode the quality of life.

Chapter Two

So You Don't Want To Die... Just Yet?

The title of this chapter had been considered as the title for the whole book, but it smacked of procrastination and, as ultimately death is inevitable, it could be tempting fate to ignore the event indefinitely.

There are circumstances when it could be most inconvenient to die, when a temporary postponement would be beneficial; such was the case recently when a pregnant woman was fatally brain damaged in a road accident but was kept 'alive' on a life-support machine until her child was born.

The difference between the phrase 'just yet' and 'a little longer' is subtle but important; the former may have practical connotations whereas the latter implies a voluntary wish. To a surprising degree the length of time that we live lies within our own control. So the words 'a little longer' are very important, not only because our lives are finite, but, more importantly, because the aggregate parts of the complex human machine have an ultimate design life of approximately 125 years. As with most complex things, there is a wealth of difference between design life and practical working life.

We will inevitably fall prey to one or more of the many diseases awaiting us as we age our way through life. Determining what malady will ultimately claim us lies to a considerable extent within our inheritance, i.e., our genes, and these lie outside our control.

We can plan to avoid, or at least postpone, many illnesses, including the more common causes of premature deaths prior to the age of 75. Apart from these there will remain the three most common 'killers' likely to be encountered after 70: those affecting the heart, cancer, dementia, or possibly all three.

Even this list, though not exhaustive, may one day be modified by promising developments in the field of biological drugs which show early promise in combating, for example, malignant melanoma, although they are unlikely to be available till the twenty-first century.

Meanwhile, for those pondering over today, the decision on which of these three might strike after 75 is not so much in the lap of the gods, as in our inheritance. A selective lifestyle will only have maximum effect on middle-age health and progressively to a lesser extent in the later years. A 'healthy' lifestyle is unlikely to have much effect on 'design faults' or 'production-line faults', which may only be rectified to a limited extent (by hip replacements or heart transplants etc.).

Osteoarthritis tends to affect older people, causing suffering through undue wear and tear and leading to a considerable deterioration in the quality of life. It may even curtail life expectation due to ensuing physical incapacity. These 'mechanical' handicaps call for resourcefulness in the sufferer, as well as doggedness and a determination to present a cheerful face to the world in spite of all evidence to the contrary; the reward lies in the admiration and help from those around.

There is another factor to be considered when weighing up how long the journey ahead might be, not just for oneself but for subsequent generations, and that means one's progeny. Should we not question the quality of life ahead for future generations? Whether there might not even be any life at all, for how far ahead can our civilisation continue with events progressing as they are? Perhaps all life might become extinct?

Before reading further, do you know how long *Homo sapiens* has existed in its present recognisable form? How does this compare with the dinosaurs' tenancy of our planet, those much-ridiculed creatures that we hold up as examples of an incapacity to thrive or survive who eventually became extinct.

A brief summary of the Earth's history will be salutary and I shall then put our own achievements, including our prospects for survival as a species, into perspective.

> *In the beginning God created the heaven and earth:*
> *And the earth was without form, and void...*
>
> Genesis 1:1–2

The question 'why not live a little longer' should not be interpreted purely as a personal one, for the viability of *Homo sapiens* as a species cannot be taken for granted and without this the question relating to future personal life becomes irrelevant and the title of the book becomes academic.

Richard Leakey and Roger Lewin in their book, *Origins Reconsidered* should be studied in order to assess the possibility of *Homo sapiens* continuing to inhabit the earth for much longer. If they are to be believed, and they forward a convincing argument, then the wisdom of propagating our species at all is brought into question.

First, the Earth's time capsule needs to be put into perspective:

4,500,000,000 years ago:	The planet Earth is created.
4,000,000,000 years ago:	Primitive life starts (in water).
430,000,000 years ago:	First (of five) mass extinctions – the Ordovician event.
350,000,000 years ago:	Primitive life on land – only to be obliterated by a second catastrophe (the Devonian).
225,000,000 years ago:	Third catastrophe strikes (the Permian).
215,000,000 years ago:	First mammals evolved, including the early dinosaurs.
200,000,000 years ago:	Fourth catastrophe (the Triassic).
65,000,000 years ago:	Fifth and most recent catastrophe (the Cretaceous). This last event extinguished some 98% of all life on earth, including the dinosaurs.

There then followed a few million relatively peaceful years allowing some of the early mammals to evolve, excluding the much-despised, but now extinct, dinosaurs. It is pertinent to register that these creatures survived in their various forms for some 160 million years (in contrast to *Homo sapiens'* mere 100,000 years to date) before the fifth catastrophe (the Cretaceous) obliterated them approximately 65 million years back, they having partially survived the fourth catastrophe.

Since that time (65 million years ago) relatively minor events have caused the significant extinction of life on earth at intervals of approximately every 26 million years, with the net result that 99% of all species that have ever lived are now extinct!

Soon after the last catastrophe (the Cretaceous), primates evolved, and...

30,000,000 years ago: First apes started.

7,500,000 years ago: *Hominids erectus.*

100,000 years ago: *Homo sapiens.*

Homo sapiens[1], amongst other distinguishing characteristics, was able to speak. The evidence for this was the occurrence on the inside of skulls of this age, of an indentation known as Broca's area, where the concept of speech is formulated. Wernicke's area is located in a similar region, and is the place where most articulation of speech originates.

Richard Leakey, in his book, *Origins Reconsidered*, puts forward a convincing argument showing that we are now in the early stages of the sixth and final mass extinction, but with two major differences to the previous five: this one is man-created, and this time there will be no recovery, in contrast to the previous five.

Evidence from fossils indicates that species of vertebrates have a longevity of approximately two million years. Leakey suggests that the next cataclysmic earthly event should not arrive for another twelve million years and on this score the prospects for *Homo sapiens* continuing for quite a while look good. However a number of things are working against this happening, not least of which are the twin threats of population and technology explosion, both of which are a form of physiological 'malignancy'.

---

[1]   *Homo sapiens sapiens* to give modern man his correct title.

There are more people (*Homo sapiens*) living today than have ever lived in the totality of man's existence. The resultant overpopulation makes the species vulnerable to extinction from, amongst other threats, the ravages of war or other forms of physical and psychological assault, which in the case of *Homo sapiens*, includes nuclear oblivion as well as disease. On this count, aggravated by overcrowding, we must anticipate the coming of a speeded-up and more sophisticated version of the AIDS virus. There is already evidence of different versions of the AIDS virus breeding in the human body and thus producing new strains.

On the subject of technology explosion, the Dutch anatomist Eugene Dubois published a paper at the beginning of the nineteenth century drawing attention to the fact that as any species has evolved, the size of the brain has doubled in size relative to the size of the body. So far this has held true for *Homo sapiens*, but man has not been content to restrict the scope and pace of his own creations so as to allow his brain's capability to expand at a commensurate pace, a pace which should have been extended over many hundreds or thousands of years, instead of over less than a century as has been the case.

Ninety per cent of man's creative products that have evolved since the wheel was invented have taken place within the last 100 years and continue to do so at an exponential rate, without brain size increasing. This has not been helped by man's impatience and restlessness, one of the spin-offs from overcrowding. These have developed technologies which have themselves hastened further advances so that man is no longer able to control them. This in turn calls for more frenzied activity to keep ahead of a science which is now rapidly getting out of control, posing a threat to man's supposed superiority.

Let us examine other species, the primates for example. The great apes (gorillas) have a brain which is far larger than is necessary for them to lead their relatively simple lifestyle; the obverse of this statement is that they have brain capability which is in reserve and unutilised. This is no longer the case in humans, we are using far too much of our reserve capability. It is as though we have drawn upon the recuperative powers generated by sleep, and instead of allowing the required 6 hours or so every 24 hours, we make ourselves do with 4 hours' sleep.

For some, this may not matter, depending on what demands are made during the waking hours, but if this level of demand were to continue indefinitely and become the norm, the central nervous system would break down. Similarly, one needs 'quiet time' (not necessarily sleep) to recuperate. For the benefit of financially orientated persons: it is as though the dividend becomes uncovered, or the borrowing ratio gets out of line, leading to 'over-trading'.

Were it not for computers, that Dickensian figure wielding a quill pen would have spotted most or all of the computer-related financial crimes occurring today, such as direct debits going berserk, or relatively junior employees removing great sums of cash from bank accounts (aided by techniques referred to as 'computer piracy', of which there are many variations, not all computer-related). Such incidents are only made possible in a 'computer-happy' society.

So what form will the coming mass extinction referred to by Leakey, take? Conflict? Disease? Starvation? Or possibly a combination of all three with massive privation accompanying a total breakdown in civilisation? Of one thing Leakey is sure: extinction is already in train and there will be no survivors. He does concede that, in the unlikely event of a regeneration, the subsequent species might, after a few million years appropriately be referred to as *Homo technologiocus*. I suspect, however, that he poses this possibility only to enable him to invent a new species by name!

How long might there be left? Again, Leakey gives a forecast on a different but relevant theme. He forecasts that 50% of today's remaining animal species will become extinct in the next 30 years. If life on Earth is finite, and imminently so, measured against the total time that the planet Earth has been in existence, then it is probably already too late to think in terms of 'lifeboat stations'. The 'ship' is already foundering, even though, as in the Titanic sinking, the orchestra is still valiantly continuing to play.

If the paleoanthropologists are to be believed, 99% of all species that have ever lived have already been exterminated by the five cataclysmic events that are known to have taken place on Earth to date. It is difficult to deny all the evidence confronting us which suggests that a sixth such event is gathering before us like a giant wave whose crest is beginning to break up before falling to engulf all before it. This time, however, in contrast to the previous cataclysmic events, it is man-induced.

What then lies ahead in the short term for the human race? How long have we left?

Perhaps the question 'why not live a little longer?' should be turned around and restated: 'don't die too soon, nor live too long'. Is the reported decrease in male sperm fertility an ominous portend? In the light of this possibility, the question of longevity might be reassessed.

Consider the last 30, 20, or even the last 10 years! What changes have taken place in our midst! The early symptoms are there to see: seventy years ago, protests became organised and took the form of 'marches'. Today the equivalent protests take the form of violence and obstructions, bringing into play masses of citizens confronting each other in the face of the increasingly inadequate forces of police, who themselves are using greater levels of physical force. This could quickly degenerate into anarchy as respect for the police and law-keepers continues to wane. Whence after that?

I suggest that the expectation of survival for the human race probably lies between 50 and 150 more years. Is this a factor to be taken into account when you consider the question, *do you still want to live a little longer?*

Perhaps it is just as well to think hard before coming to a definite conclusion, as the quality of life at the far end comes increasingly into question.

The Ultimate Weapon

I have suggested that the human race might become extinct within 50–150 years. I felt that had I pursued this possibility, there was a risk that this book might have been consigned to the flames, but that would have been akin to sweeping dust under the carpet. The reason I now return to this theme is that the Ebola virus outbreak in Africa was successfully contained (not suppressed), and retreated back to lurk in the forests whence it came. There are, however, other viruses (Marburg is one, and every bit as dangerous as Ebola), which doubtless await their opportunity.

As we have observed, the next and sixth (final, in Leakey's opinion) cataclysmic event to strike the planet Earth could be man-induced, and there is gathering evidence indicating that viruses could be the very threat to trigger off the catastrophe.

In parallel with viruses, man is not helping himself by having allowed overcrowding to explode, with not just more people per unit area of Earth's surface, but more aggressive movement further, faster, more often, and under more crowded conditions, all of which aid the spread of infections including viruses. The overcrowding threat is even compounded by details such as passenger aircraft cabin air now being changed less frequently in the name of economy. The result is that we inhale our fellow passengers' exhaled and infected air in a more concentrated form and more frequently.

How long is it since you had a cold? Whatever your age, it is more than likely that it was followed by a chest infection or laryngitis or maybe even the feeling of being 'just off colour'. The odds are that you were given antibiotics, which probably did not hasten your recovery. You may have been concerned at how 'run down' you were, for the 'infection' seemed to drag on and on, accompanied by inexplicable lethargy. Meanwhile, the conventional bacteria are becoming increasingly resistant to repeated doses of antibiotics. Perhaps you feel that antibiotics cause symptoms which make you averse to taking them at all. If these incidents only affected the older generation then one might put them down to ageing, but all ages are affected.

There are many variants of viruses just awaiting the opportunity to be picked up. We should be thankful that the Ebola and Marburg viruses kill so quickly, before, as with AIDS, the infected person has had opportunities to pass them on rather like a chain letter.

Let us examine what Mother Nature could have up her secret sleeve, and draw up an ideal specification for a real killer virus capable of wiping out *Homo sapiens*.

1) The virus should be capable of lying dormant for a long time, millions of years if necessary (prehistoric wasps have been demonstrated to be holding viruses).

2) It should be able to survive extreme conditions (the tubercle bacillus can do this).

3) It should not kill too quickly so that the infected person has time to pass the infection on to as many others as possible. Thus far AIDS has been remarkably successful in this respect, with an incubation period that is measured in years rather than days. It does not

disclose its presence overtly even during this lengthy incubation period.

4) It should be capable of mutation within the host.

5) It should possess 'radar jamming' so as to throw the host's defences off the trail through mutation.

6) Perhaps the most desirable characteristic is to be able to be borne in droplets, so that the spread is similar to that of the common cold. Once this state has been reached, the human race may well be doomed.

Alternatively the virus should be able to have a 'jump-ride' through insects (like mosquitoes and flies) and so infect a wider sphere of humans. It might be later than we think!

And so much for the probable, or even possible, viruses of the future. Are we yet sure that a virus will be the vehicle of our final demise after a mere 100,000 years' struggle?

Mother Nature meanwhile relentlessly continues to search for the ultimate destructive weapon and we are unwittingly aiding and abetting her, rather than preparing adequate defences. The reverse, in fact, as, instead of husbanding defensive characteristics such as humility, privacy and discipline (including sufficiently severe degrees of punishment to deter offenders), the human race is exposing itself to every threat that nature might deploy.

A prime and recent example is Bovine Spongiform Encephalopathy (BSE) and its associated publicity stablemate Creutzfeldt-Jakob disease (CJD). Though the link between these two diseases is largely tenuous, and as yet unproven as a serious threat to mankind's survival, the secondary threat is to man's economic stability. The consequences of political and media hysteria can only be wondered at and the question pondered as to whether the term 'mad' has been correctly apportioned. Rather, the whole topic of mankind's stability must surely be brought into question along with that of whether he is capable of wielding the 'weapons' of mass communication safely and in an uncensored manner?

Under a combined onslaught of fear and ignorance, and hyped by media publicity, a dearth of political leadership is uncovered and politicians are exposed for all their ineptitude. Though it may be politically unacceptable, it would be more sensible from a health standpoint to ban all imports of tobacco (amongst other things) and leave the choice of consuming beef to individuals in the light of the evidence as it is revealed.

I would like to add an opinion to the weight of that already forwarded, and this relates to the future of BSE. Though still at an early stage of the story, if I am correct, BSE will not be remembered by many in five years' time (like the salmonella panic on which pyre Edwina Currie lost credibility but gained notoriety); if I am wrong, I will have had the satisfaction of having enjoyed my roast beef for many years.

Of more serious import for mankind's survival is the decline of confidence in our political leaders who have been found wanting and can only encourage contempt for authority, a prerequisite for anarchy.

Meanwhile, it should not be assumed that the terminal threat to the continuing survival of *Homo sapiens* comes from other animal species, or for that matter from any one particular source. It comes from any number of sources amongst which can be counted:

1) Disease – either bacterial in character, or gene-inspired.
2) Overpopulation leading to overcrowding, not only in the physical sense.
3) Nuclear disaster, including weaponry.
4) Mutual mass destruction, preceded by anarchy.
5) Extraterrestrial event, which is unlikely for 12 million years.

Contributory factors:

a) Greed, including argentosis. (See Chapter VII.)
b) Lack of privacy (including official technological intrusion).
c) Decline of mutual consideration (manners).
d) Inability to keep abreast with technological advances.
e) Proliferation of mental crises (emotional breakdown).

All the above factors are mentioned in different parts of this book.

Like the portent of a gathering storm, many of the early warnings of the coming disaster are already visible. It is significant that homicide rates have risen much more dramatically in 'developed' countries than 'undeveloped' countries.

Chapter Three
Death

The very word smacks of finality. This was impressed upon me at the annual Service of Dedication for the Order of St John held in St Paul's Cathedral. At one point in the service, the banners of all those senior knights who have passed away during the preceding year are solemnly paraded up to the altar, folded up and sealed in metal caskets. This ceremony marks the end.

Perhaps because of the sombre finality and associated apprehension for those left behind, many people seek solace in the conviction that this event does not mark the end, but merely the beginning. It is not the purpose of this book to put the case either for or against life after death, but rather life before death, but it did seem to justify researching the subject of death, albeit unsatisfactorily, at the outset, rather than leaving it to the end of the book.

Hence the chapter on death is one of the earliest in this book, and perhaps by including it this early I might be seeking atonement for my own knowledge (or lack of it) on this particular subject. The more research I did, the more elusive and less tangible the subject became.

I have been involved in the field of research, mostly medical, in life, amongst subjects as varied as aviation medicine, industrial medicine, road traffic accidents (a major cause of death), first aid (a prophylactic against death) and other phlegmatic subjects, but death is paradoxically the most elusive. Nobody with personal experience of death is available for consultation, for there are no survivors. I exclude those who have had a theoretical 'death', as the definition is suspect.

I began my research by tracking down alleged experiences of people who claimed to have 'died', and were able to describe the manner of their 'death', but there was always a flaw.

For example, there was the story of the man who was attending Mass in a cathedral on a warm day. Overcome by the heat during the sermon he leaned forward, buried his head in his hands and fell asleep. When the next phase of the service began, this man was dreaming and his dream took on the nightmarish quality of his being led to the guillotine where his head was placed on the block. The verger, seeing that he had fallen asleep came and tapped him on the back of his neck at the very moment when, in his dream, the guillotine knife descended and chopped his head off. The shock of all this was that he suffered a fatal heart attack and never regained consciousness.

The other story, also apocryphal, concerns a merchant who lived 2500 years ago, in the Arabian desert. Returning home at the end of a tiring day, he tethered his camel and approached his front door. He was contemplating how many years he might have to live, when, on opening his front door, he was horrified to find a spectral figure lurking in the dark interior. The spectre spoke in a synthesised voice.

"Welcome home on one of your last visits – I represent my company, Death Release. I carry a message from my chairman, and as the messenger of Death I am to tell you that we have an appointment in the near future."

The merchant, aghast, slammed the door shut, ran to his second camel; gathered himself together, throwing a harness over the beast's head before mounting, and proceeded to beat the animal into a fast trot over the desert. He continued thus all night and into the following day, to get as far as possible from his frightening encounter with his destiny.

As the sun began to rise, he came across an oasis which showed signs of habitation, and, having tethered his camel, he staggered to the heavy wooden door of the local hostelry, where he knocked frantically as the first of the rising sun's rays lit up the entrance. As the heavy door opened, creaking on its rusty hinges, he was able to make out a form inside, lit by the first rays of the rising sun, an eerie figure, which beckoned him inside with what passed for a welcome, holding out both arms to help the traveller over the threshold, but all the traveller could see was the spectre of death. As the by now terrified merchant sank to the floor, the 'spectre' extended his arms to catch the falling body. As the merchant lost consciousness for the last time, he heard the voice saying, "I thought you were never coming." The inn-keeper, dressed in a white nightshirt, had waited up all night for his last guest. He gazed at the motionless figure on the floor as he muttered, "This is not the guest I was expecting, and I fear he is dead."

The more I attempted to investigate 'death' the more unsatisfactory the subject became. There were many and varied stories about people who had 'died' and returned to the living world. The experiences they had to recount were varied, but seemed to have one theme in common: the people concerned told tales of how 'my whole life was laid out before me' or 'I seemed to be floating' or 'I entered into a world of heavenly light'. The more I learned about these tales, the more they seemed to share something – a dream.

My conclusion was to question the whole definition of death. Perhaps the goalposts need realigning. Perhaps clinical death needed to have a time factor added, such as the patient being clinically dead (i.e. heart and breathing stopped) for, say, five minutes, by which time there would be irreversible brain stem death in addition. If this were to be accepted, then a brief crossing of the present threshold (no heartbeat) would be compatible with a dream. Perhaps the sleep equivalent of the REM (rapid eye movements), when dreams and fantasises materialise, would be the nearest one might come to the actual experience of dying.

Such a hypothesis would neatly explain how, with the onset of old age, when geriatrics tend to doze off very easily and repeatedly, a limbo stage of the twilight world is inhabited. During this stage, the subject is neither asleep properly (though his eyes are closed), nor truly awake, but floating in a fantasy world where thoughts wander around the semi-conscious mind. A similar state is induced by inhaling nitrous oxide (laughing gas) which is used as a light anaesthetic. During the recovery phase, the real secret of the universe suddenly appears to be at one's fingertips, only to slip away as full consciousness returns. It is possible that older persons go through repeated mini-deaths, or lead-ins to them, as though in preparation for the real, ultimate death experience!

The biggest obstacle for me was that nobody existed with practical experience of real death, or, to be precise, was available to recount their experience. I turned to the literature on the subject of death, but this was no more helpful than the literature on unidentified flying objects, all full of enthusiasm but nothing totally credible.

I examined Margot Grey's researches in her book *Return from Death*, in which she interviewed people who had allegedly returned from the other side, but found it 'unsatisfactory and unsafe' (in legal terminology). Whilst very much respecting her views, I was not wholly convinced that her subjects had actually died, but rather believed that they had ventured too close to the precipice, before turning back having had a fright. Perhaps their experience was akin to a dream state, accentuated by auto-suggestion in the circumstances of a near-death situation.

Dr Frances Kampler in her researches (*Ghosts, Visions And Voices*) had some logical explanations for psychic experiences relating to death and near-death experiences. There is little doubt that as one gets older and more prone to oxygen deprivation to the brain, caused by innumerable transient arterial shortcomings, then hallucinatory-type incidents occur. These are especially likely to happen in later years as 'waking dreams', which occur during the 'clouded conscious' stages of waking up or falling asleep. These are the breeding grounds for ghosts and similar hallucinatory experiences to take root. They are not, however, confined to the elderly, but can, and do, happen at any age. Anybody who has suffered from sleep deprivation, i.e., been awake for 24 hours or longer, and has experienced 'mind wandering' with hallucinatory experiences as a result, will understand. Illness can also precipitate such experiences, which can be associated with toxaemia, medication or raised body temperature, and can be especially dangerous when, for example, driving, or when any decision-taking is required; this is another reason for being aware of jet lag, especially as self-awareness is also impaired.

If we define 'legal death' as being the state of being clinically dead for five minutes, this would re-categorise those at present termed as 'having died' into those who had 'lapsed into unconsciousness', and their stories into 'dreams'. I became aware though that such a move might well have legal (mis)interpretations, for when I mentioned this to a lawyer one day his eyes gleamed (I could see him identifying a new and lucrative source of income).

By contrast I found Mrs Elizabeth Kubler-Ross and *Death - The Final Stage Of Growth* more encouraging in that she approached death as being the natural finality of *living*, stressing the importance of living one's life to the full. Her approach left one with the feeling that dying was akin to drawing the bedroom curtains before what was finally going to be an extended sleep and that what happened afterwards was of little consequence.

The precise timing of death can be influenced by the patient within quite large time scales. I knew of a mother who had been suffering from a particularly virulent form of cancer for many years, during which time she had had a hindquarter amputation (her leg was amputated at hip level). She had a daughter who suffered from a form of depression with a well-defined cycle which could be predicted. This daughter was close to her mother and depended heavily on her support, especially during the acute phase of her illness. As the mother was clearly getting near the end of her life, the girl was in the middle of a depressive phase, and the mother stated that she would not go until her daughter had emerged from her depression. She achieved this and then stopped eating and within days she was entering the dying phase of her illness. Her husband, an eminent physician of no particularly strong religious persuasion, was at her bedside, and as she slipped away holding his hand, he found the experience so moving that he said he was certain that God was holding her other hand. He said that he will treasure this memory for ever.

As the final hours of life ebb away, my conclusions from watching many in this situation is that it is akin to twilight sleep and it is no coincidence that as people become older they tend to slip into this penumbral state increasingly easily and more frequently, as though preparing their bodies for something. Unlike sleep, however, their dreams become less vivid and more tranquil.

On a lighter note, Mark Twain's oft-quoted cable, 'The report of my death was an exaggeration', is not unique. A friend of mine, John Hoggard, who is very much enjoying life in Sussex, England, still relishes his own experience. As a sub lieutenant in the Royal Navy, he was serving in an armed merchant cruiser in the Second World War, when his ship was sunk. He was reported in *The Times* as 'missing believed killed', and his mother received a letter from his former housemaster at King's School, Worcester, offering condolences. By this time, the casualty list had been amended to 'Sub Lieutenant Hoggard now POW', giving his number and camp (it was Colditz and according to John – 'not nearly as frugal as my public school!') as given to the Red Cross.

After John was released at the end of the war, he noticed in his school magazine a photograph of the war memorial in college hall, with his own name engraved on a centre panel. He at once wrote to the school authorities, giving them the good tidings that he was clinically alive, and suggesting that they had been a bit hasty, and giving his permission for his name to be removed from the 'THEY DIED FOR ENGLAND' memorial.

Psychological Deprivation (PD)

It may sound daunting, but this subtitle marks the switch from death back to the living, although one sufferer from PD described it as a 'living hell'. The prime target of this book is life in preference perhaps to death and all the finality that the word implies.

Having turned my attention to the other side of the great divide, and paused briefly halfway as I did so, I now returned to those who are left behind, in order that I might obtain the views of those who begin the journey towards the final chapters with their loved ones, but who turn back at the exit. I recalled how I had on many occasions visited terminally ill patients who begged me not to divulge the terminal nature of their illnesses to their partners, only to be told in turn by their partner not to inform the patient of the seriousness of their illness. It was in such a situation that one felt that the practice of true medicine had so much in common with the priesthood, and the bringing together of such a couple for their final days together was almost beyond earthly understanding.

Similarly, nurses have an insight and understanding which is almost on the extrasensory perception level. I recall a man dying of cancer who, near the end, was in bed and by now unconscious; his wife was holding his hand, when the nurse quietly took her arm and said that it was time to leave. What she really meant was that it time for *him* to leave and that his wife was detaining him. Sure enough, as soon as his hand was released he left, for where I am not sure, but he was no longer with us. It was as though a ship had slipped its moorings, and within a few moments he had left, quietly, as though the very fact of having his hand held had acted like a mooring rope preventing his departure.

One optimist pointed out that the initials PD took priority over PM (post-mortem). In his optimistic way he added, "Even if I have halitosis, bad breath is infinitely better than no breath at all."

Causes of Psychological Deprivation

1) Death of a loved one.

2) Divorce: whether caused by absence of love or even unrequited love.

3) Partings, be they permanent or temporary.

4) Change of location.

5) Change of circumstances, e.g., financial, social, or even work-related.

6) Change in health.

7) Disappointment: failed ambition or expectations in relationships.

Effects of Psychological Deprivation

Symptoms range from grieving, in the first case, across the whole spectrum of psychological illness, from mild sadness, frustration, insomnia, uncontrollable restlessness, frenetic activity, 'heartache', self-torment intermingled with passion (anger or resentment), 'disagreeableness' or irritability, melancholia, leading to physical illness, anorexia, and even suicide.

The whole syndrome can be summarised in one word: STRESS.

Returning to the causes of PD:

1) *Grieving*, except in the case of sudden death, begins a long time before the actual event in that it has to be prepared for. When death comes, grieving is all-important for the survivor, for it is a very natural act, a form of rehabilitation, and it is essential for it to take its time, for it cannot be hurried. As a rule of thumb, every anniversary has to be experienced before grieving can be said to have run its initial course. During this time, few, if any, decisions affecting lifestyle should be taken, for in the stage of shock it is easy to make the wrong decision.

Even after the initial year there remains a further period (lasting up to a further three years, I would suggest, from my personal observations of several hundred cases) before the topic of a departed close one can be discussed easily. All the more reason why no major decisions should be taken for at least two years, if they can be deferred. Grieving is not only confined to the acute emotionally painful phase. Like a wound, it can leave a scar after apparent healing has taken place and, like a scar, can give rise to unexpected twinges.

Convalescence following a period of grief is affected by age (and relative age), by the comparability and closeness of the parties, by independence of the survivor and, most importantly the availability of outside support.

One striking factor marks grief from all other non-lethal events: the prognosis is usually hopeful (time being 'a good healer'), unlike divorce, where ongoing and recurring problems and stimuli tend to hinder recovery. There may also be an additional healing factor in a sense of release from suffering which enables relief to replace regret, regret which can remain after divorce.

The essential factor about death is that it is final. There is no escape, no going back, no option but to take the future as it comes. This has certain advantages in that nothing is left except memories. These are progressively subjugated as new experiences are superimposed upon those of the past, and the healing process steadily proceeds in much the same way as a wound heals over. So the grief ebbs, allowing a new form, a soothing cloak, to take its place. It is important to allow oneself to become enveloped in this cloak, for it is a form of medication akin to a wound dressing.

2) *Divorce*. Grieving is not confined to death; a form of grief can be caused by other terminal situations, such as a parting, either from a person or from a location, as when one leaves home. In either case, it may be temporary or permanent with diverse consequences.

If the event is of a temporary nature then the 'recovery' will probably be straightforward, with the added benefit of providing an immunity to subsequent episodes. If permanent, as when moving to a new location, the compensating advantages tend to minimise the trauma felt.

If caused by the break-up of a family, as in the case of divorce, the stress and grief caused is likely to be considerable, especially if one party did not wish for divorce, and particularly if (as in the case of parents) one sees one's children suffering; the chances are that one is not privy to the full causes that bring such misery about.

What then are the differences, if any, in the type of grief caused by parting caused by death, and a parting caused by divorce?

In the case of divorce, where emotions will have played a part (for emotions are an essential ingredient), different circumstances prevail to those of a death, circumstances which are ongoing and delay the essential healing taking place, thus delaying recovery. More permanent damage can be caused by family break-up than by a death.

It is no coincidence that divorces rarely happen between persons after they have reached 70, for there is a lack of the emotional fuel so essential for animosity to flourish. Perhaps psychiatrists might have a part to play in reducing the number of divorces, except that they are themselves suspect, for they seem to become 'programmed' by contact with their patients!

An interesting by-product of the high incidence of divorces (one in every three marriages) is the large number of unattached, relatively young men and women with unrequited needs, 'peripatetic threats to my security' as one middle-aged, but rapidly ageing woman once put it to me. Their 'hunting habits' are to be seen in the modern versions of agony columns in quite respectable papers.

One such notice showed originality, if not desperation in its appeal – 'Presentable elderly gentleman would like to meet suitable lady to enjoy the autumn of his life – before the leaves fall off.'

3) *Partings* are a more acute form of PD, and are usually self-limiting, though none the less painful in the moment.

4) *Change of location* can be a cause of 'homesickness' if a parting is involved, but does not usually give rise to long-term problems.

5) *Deterioration in health* and

6) *Disappointment* can cause 'pangs', and is only a mild form of PD that does not call for anything other than a passing mention. In certain circumstances, disappointment can be a cause of chronic grief, as when a career is terminated, possibly due to health or financial constraint.

Animals and Death

Are animals aware of death? Certainly they are, in so far as self-preservation is concerned. Like *Homo sapiens* they are also aware of impending death for themselves as individuals and know when 'their time is near'. They will seek a suitable place or location where they might pass their final hours.

So far as their own kind is concerned, animals would not always seem to be unduly aware of impending death nor always take more than a passing interest when it happens, though there are exceptions. Grief, as we know it, appears to take a different form in the animal kingdom, at least superficially. Certain breeds (swans are an example) mate for life and it is difficult to know or identify in human terms what form the grief takes when a mate is lost, except that it is 'different'.

In the canine world, the loss of a master can precipitate widely different 'feelings' of loss. At one extreme, a devoted dog will stay with his dying master, even protecting his body after the death. At the other extreme, I can recall a dog so devoted to his master that he insisted on accompanying him on all occasions. Yet when his master suddenly dropped down dead of a coronary and the dog was shown the body, he took one perfunctory sniff, metaphorically shrugged his tail, and turned away, transferring his devotion to his master's widow. Within a few days, the dog's daily routine had taken the form of 'devotion to mistress'.

At both extremes it appears that animals recognise the significance and consequences of death, taking a pragmatic view and resuming what life still has to offer in a most practical manner.

Chapter Four
Meet Your Cremator

O Death, where is thy sting?
O Grave where is thy victory?

First Epistle of Paul to the Corinthians 16:55

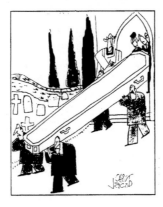

"God knows how long we've been metric, but that casket maker still hasn't got the hang of it."

Following the examination of death at the beginning of this book, in preference to the more usual place for death to be, the finish, this chapter will talk about life.

Death is a paradox. Many persons during life may well have gone about guarding their financial affairs with a high degree of secrecy, like a squirrel hiding its nuts, without apparently remembering that soon after death financial details of their estate would be publicly available. Details of one's financial status, as seen by the Inland Revenue, are registered for anyone who might wish to find out. They are also widely advertised in the newspapers.

Death is an enigma, and finally has to be taken as it comes, though everyone has some, but only some say in how, when, and even to some degree, what form it takes.

The experience of living and dying might be compared to parachuting, in that once the parachutist has left the aircraft, his arrival back to earth is inevitable, though the exact method of arrival, e.g., how soon, speed of impact, location, degree of pain incurred, is to a considerable and, one might add, a surprising degree under one's own volition, for there is a considerable amount of control available with which to determine the end, inevitable though that end might be.

Accountants make a living and, some might add, not an inconsiderable fortune from advising on taxes. Why then should there not be a living for suitably inclined specialists in the art of dying? Why should death not therefore be considered as an art? Some of the mystique and even fear might then be removed from the aura surrounding the subject. If not a fortune, then is there a living to be made from death? Indeed there is, and some professions do. The best known are undertakers, who are professional mourners and only look serious when they are acting in that role. They are, if anything, jollier persons in real life than their fellow beings. Why? Possibly because they have come to terms with the very subject of death. Maybe it is a compensatory stance, or maybe they are just realists. "It's just an everyday occurrence," as one cheerfully put it.

The 'sting' of death might well be worse in the anticipation than the event, so the more it can be contemplated and assessed the easier it is to set the whole subject aside and get on with the usually enjoyable task of living. The purpose of this chapter, therefore, is to do just that, so that the remainder of the book might be devoted to more pressing matters such as savouring the enjoyments of what is available in living. Therefore, consider the subject diligently; decide what one is able or unable to do to vary the inevitability, and then get on with what remains in the real world of living. There are many modern day examples of people who have become obsessed with the subject and squandered the immediate joys of being alive; the aircraft designer Howard Hughes is an example of 'head-in-sand' (or perhaps 'body-in-mortuary') mentality. Genius though he was, he became obsessive about life-threatening infections, and for practical purposes 'died by isolation' many years prematurely. It is the mentality of going to catch an aircraft flight several days before the actual departure date in case it is missed.

The Undertaker

Undertakers, consultants in death, as I once heard them described, are essential members of the community. They have been likened to human scavengers, but they do provide an important garbage-disposal service. Like the judiciary, they prefer to wear a disguise (sombre suits, funereal gait, grim expression), but, unlike the judiciary, no wig, but a top hat, so that they are not recognised when they resume their rightful place in the daily social round. When it comes to discussing their professional life they are quite realistic about their responsibilities, which are not inconsiderable.

Their services are called upon when a family's morale is at a low ebb, and is in no state to question cost or value for money; in a situation which is about as infrequent for the average family as buying a house, though without, in the latter case, having time to think much about it and with even less inclination to pick and choose. Undertakers' charges are not usually questioned, and trust is all implicit. 'Best buy' is not appropriate.

An undertaker's overheads are not inconsiderable.

"Have you ever considered," an undertaker said to me, as I watched him polishing his hearse (I had been called to see him as he was suffering from tenosynovitis, due to overzeal in preparing the vehicle for its 'next run', as he put it), "what driving around at 15 m.p.h. does to an engine? Cars are like humans, you know, they need exercise; the last time this hearse went over 35 m.p.h. was because we were going to 'miss our slot' at the crematorium.

"Only collected one ticket for speeding," he reflected. "I accelerated through some lights to try and get the whole cortège through in one go, and the police were waiting with their radar: most degrading it was – we all had to stop of course, and for a moment I thought they were going to issue a multiple ticket. I tried to persuade them to issue the ticket in the name of the deceased, but they wouldn't hear of it. However, after a form of plea bargaining, they agreed to issue only one ticket instead of tickets for six individual cars. It had to be me, of course, and I tried to plead special circumstances, but the court was not sympathetic. However, I'll get my revenge eventually – I've made a special note of who was sitting on the bench that day.

"Another thing which people do not appreciate," he continued, "is that these crematoriums [*sic*] are not the same as the traditional graveyard services where there is a healing atmosphere. It's those bloody accountants that have got into the act, they are all for turnover, and they run crematoriums [*sic*] like supermarkets. I once heard an accountant doing a 'time and motion' study at a crematorium, and suggesting that the curtain could be speeded up a bit, and so get an extra customer dealt with."

He continued, "Have you ever thought about the quality control required at a crematorium? I mean the wood for the coffins. It has to have just the right combustibility, and this, together with the mixture control, will determine whether visible smoke comes out of the chimney or not, and this upsets the next customer."

He was clearly in an expansive mood, so I let him go on.

"Life is not what it used to be; I heard of a chap the other day, whom I'd been watching keenly for a while, and bless my soul, when he died it emerged that he had got planning permission to dig his own grave on his own land. I thought of putting in an appeal, as a ratepayer, but I reckoned that that would have complicated matters too much so I settled for dropping a card through the letter box, saying if there was anything I could do to help... As it happened I got the job but at a much-reduced rate."

At that moment a rival's hearse passed by.

"See that fellow? Now there's a keen businessman. Name's Mortimer, is known in the business as Mortis for short. Over-keen if you ask me. Got pinched for speeding a couple of months ago, when he tried to fit in too many customers during the flu epidemic, but now we always try to help one another out in busy times, which for some reason usually happens when there is a full moon. I once suggested to Mort that we might introduce a reciprocal trade arrangement between us, but he caught me going into the doctor's surgery and reckoned he would be on to a loser, though he did say that he would offer my family a discount of ten per cent when my time comes.

"No, trade is not good nowadays. My turnover was down 5% last year, but that was better than the national average; overall deaths were down from 660,000 in 1991, to 600,000 in 1992, but it can't last. Two good summers (I hate good weather) were to blame; also these geriatric homes are not helping – too much central heating! But it's a bit like the builders' land bank, the logjam will break soon. There are now over 2,300 people alive today, all over 100 years of age. No wonder they cancelled telegrams – the Queen just couldn't afford to keep it up! But death rates are bound to return to normal soon, though meanwhile this competition is ruinous. Did you know that the cost of the average funeral today is just three times the average weekly wage, compared with about nine times fifty years ago?

"Every now and then we get a bonus. In January 1997 there were 10,000 extra deaths, thanks entirely to the Asian flu epidemic. We had to double up, putting two bodies into a single refrigerated slot until we caught up with ourselves. However, the cemetery land bank is running out; I see that legislation is being drawn up to allow old corpses to be dug up after twenty-five years to make room for newcomers. Anyway the majority of people dying today opt for cremation. I've thought about approaching my Member of Parliament with a view to introducing a Private Member's Bill making an option for cremation compulsory in the small print of wills, but he hasn't been looking too well of late and I reckoned that he might have had to declare an imminent interest in the subject matter. I'll keep an eye on him though... one never knows.

"As for marketing funerals, I watch the trends in supermarkets, like special offers, but the difficulty is that although coffins are not always 'made to measure', though we try and persuade our customers that they are, any advance order is likely to lead to trouble, for a terminal illness can wreak havoc with body measurements taken too far in advance. I remember a twenty-two-stone chap, looked very ill, I reckoned, and I would have bet a fiver that he would be gone within a couple of weeks; so, with an eye to getting the business, I made up an outsize coffin."

"What happened? A bright, young, newly qualified locum came on the scene and talked him into losing some weight, and, burn my timbers, he recovered, leaving me with an outsize coffin with nothing to put into it. What can you do? One can hardly advertise an 'end-of-season sale', it would not be appropriate – even 'cancelled order' might raise suspicions. Finally I got rid of it as a 'special offer', but when it came to the funeral the customer was much smaller than I had been led to believe, and the corpse rattled around inside like a pea in a pod. That, however, was not the end of the story, for the pall-bearers were of an uneven height, and when the occupant slid from one end to the other going up the church steps, too much weight fell on the smallest pall-bearer, who slipped on some of the flowers as they fell off the coffin, and he uttered an oath which was fortunately muffled when the organist inadvertently pressed the fortissimo stop. With hindsight, I should have cut my losses and chopped the damned thing up for firewood, which at least would have had the merit of being used for a similar purpose to that originally envisaged."

"Yes, there have been some near misses; perhaps the greatest disappointment in my life was that my daughter became engaged to an orthopaedic surgeon. I believe he was attracted by the fact that he was told that his prospective father-in-law owned six Rolls Royces, and it wasn't until after the engagement was announced that he discovered they were all hearses!

"I think the final blow came when he found me reading the daily paper with a pencil in my hand. He believed I was doing the crossword puzzle, and he looked askance when I explained I was simply carrying out some essential market research: going through the 'deaths', and comparing these figures with my sales ledger, for I always prided myself on catching forty-five per cent of the market.

"Sadly, this budding surgeon explained that he didn't feel altogether happy at the prospect of marrying an undertaker's daughter, in case the idea got around that we were aiming at a sort of 'one stop service', from the table to the grave, which, although it might be good for my business, might not be altogether beneficial for his. A pity in many ways, but perhaps it has turned out for the best in the end, for she is now married to a solicitor who specialises in drawing up wills. I believe they now offer a 'package' including a discount on the funeral. Anyway, it's a safer way to earn a living than being a member of the 'we-have-ignition' crowd."

I asked him what he meant – was it something to do with 'lift-off' and possibly destination 'space'?

He replied, "You know who I mean, the 'dust-to-instant-dust' crowd."

I suddenly realised what he was talking about: crematoria, with whom there might clearly be a potential conflict of interests.

I asked a man who owned a chain of crematoria as to what the possible implication of the suggestion that there could be 'death after death' was in his business. He knew what I meant at once and, feeling inside his jacket pocket, produced a scrumpled piece of paper, which I realised had been torn from the *British Medical Journal*. My new-found friend explained that the medical article described how the Health and Safety Executive had been investigating health and working conditions at crematoria. In the course of their researches they realised that they had uncovered a hitherto unsuspected, and unusual source of metal poisoning, as well as dioxin poisoning, from corpses in crematoria!

These poisonous substances were given off from customers when their body temperatures rose significantly to about 1000 degrees Centigrade. In the course of his investigations, the author of the article found at some twenty crematoria a wide variety of articles amongst the residual 'dust' which was all that was left after cremation. These included many types of metal objects such as hip and knee joints, screws (used in brain and central nervous system operations, sliding hip screws, a substantial number of coins (associated with various ethnic social customs), and surprisingly, a wide selection of surgical forceps; also a pacemaker, a micrometer and a pair of Mayo scissors.

To justify the investigation, the health and safety board swiftly introduced new guidelines whereby the temperature of the furnace is required to be even higher than hitherto; the reason for this is not immediately apparent, but it is known that the furnace wall is going to have to be reinforced, so a moratorium (perhaps an unfortunate choice of words) is to be made until the turn of the century.

It is also estimated that 72% of all bodies will be required to be examined and issued with a medical certificate to show that they have been freed from 'dangerous substances' before being consigned to the fires. Maybe death is not so final after all! It is understood that the choice of words on this new medical certificate has yet to be determined.

We will be considering the possibilities of the options open to us in choosing the way of death later, but if the way of dying has already disclosed itself then the timing of the end can still, within limits, be varied. So much for the final timing when you have held out until the very end. There exist a number of choices long before this point has been reached, and we shall consider some of the options of which this ultimate option, voluntary euthanasia, is one. Meanwhile, the task of continuing life should prevail.

There is little doubt that exercise has an important part to play in the promotion of general well-being, though its place in the actual prolongation of life is open to some question, but will be discussed elsewhere in this book. Jogging is a common, if somewhat artificial way of exercising, but I have been somewhat discouraged from indulging in this by the all too frequent sudden deaths which seem to overtake those who are to be seen puffing around our public parks and lanes. Furthermore, I have never seen a jogger smile, much less look happy. In fact, they give the impression that they are contemplating the worst.

Death should be treated like a daily bowel movement, or, should we say, the reverse, in that if it doesn't happen then one can score a health point. Either way, as a topic it should be considered periodically, and one's affairs should be kept in order or reviewed and then the career of living pursued with vigour.

Chapter Five
A Visit to the Tax Inspector

*In this world nothing can be said to be certain, except Death
and taxes.*

Benjamin Franklin (1706–1790)

Benjamin Franklin's dictum made an examination of the subject of
taxes mandatory in any study of death. The two subjects are
intertwined as ivy is with the tree upon which it grows.

For though death brings relief from mortal pain, such is not the
case for taxes, but rather the reverse, for taxation, far from relaxing
its grip, brings new forms of tyranny into play. Once termed 'death
duties' this macabre-sounding term has now been replaced by the
milder-sounding 'inheritance tax'.

I once asked a tax inspector, why 'inheritance tax'? Surely it was
a little late for the deceased to inherit anything and possibly 'residual
tax' might have been more descriptive? He gently explained to me
that inheritance tax had seemed a more appropriate term to the
commissioners, as all inspectors were briefed to 'inherit' as much of
an estate as could be justified for the treasury, who would be the
main beneficiary!

Such then are the macabre, even vulture-like characteristics of
that part of the Treasury which handles estates before granting
probate. Being concerned for the living as we are, we need only
confine our interest to those tax inspectors who handle day-to-day
taxation matters. Being predatorial by training, if not by nature,
their activities provoke a good deal of stress, in itself threatening our
stated objective, living 'a little longer'. A little understanding of the
territory on which tax inspectors might be found grazing could
therefore be instructive and could even prevent the more harmful
effects of stress.

One of the first facts to be learned is that, in contrast to most other channels in life, that fine fall-back, a sense of humour, is completely lacking in the tax inspector.

I once received a 'demand' for 6p. At first I thought it must be a joke, so I ignored it. I was swiftly made to realise that the word 'joke' was an unknown entity in the tax machinery dictionary, for a red-coloured follow-up demand swiftly arrived, couched in dire terms about 'collecting interest' if I failed to pay by whatever extended date had been worked out. As I understand it, interest does not accrue below a stated fixed amount owed. I thought for just one moment that this might be what could pass for a joke in government circles. The next sentence dispersed any such thought, as terms like 'distress' were used, coupled with a veiled reference to possible imprisonment etc.

I collected a postal order (the cost of which outweighed the tax demand), put a stamp on the envelope, and despatched it, together with a request ('please') for a receipt, which duly came. I still have this 'valuable' document, framed.

There followed several years of comparative silence except for periodic exchanges of the annual tax return, and though I sent this in regularly, I never seemed to have an acknowledgement, which should have given rise to concern, for my 'employment' had become somewhat complicated due to a variety of part-time sources of income, including some writing.

One morning, to my consternation, I received a letter addressed personally to me at home posing some complicated questions and suggesting that 'there might be something missing' and would I 'like to discuss it' and pay a visit to the local tax inspector's office.

All most worrying, and I searched my memory as to what might be implied. It felt like the Inland Revenue's equivalent of 'helping police with their enquiries' and it certainly made me feel jittery, and I was beginning to suffer from insomnia. How should I handle this situation? Should I treat it like going to confession, or should I employ a high-charging accountant to accompany me?

Whichever line I might choose, the implication was that my tax affairs were in a right old mess and I was in for a difficult time. By this time I was convinced I had developed a stomach ulcer, and, fearing the worst, I made an appointment to call at my local tax office.

A visit to the local tax office is an experience which everyone should savour at least once, for although tax inspectors give the impression of being de-humanised, or 'programmed' as one computer expert put it, before they are released on the public at large, they turn into human beings when cornered, as the following story reveals. On reflection, 'released' is not an appropriate word, for these souls are sentenced to spend the rest of their natural working lives like troglodytes in offices that must surely make Wormwood Scrubs seem like a five-star hotel. The mentality is conditioned to match. Though I was unable to put my reasoning into words I was reminded of those wretched beagle dogs who were conditioned into being chain smokers in exchange for their daily food. Only once did I meet a tax inspector outside his office and that was when I visited him on his deathbed. Trying to be friendly, I entered into a conversation about his life, at which he stiffened and said that it was no business of mine. The only thing that mattered was whether I had paid the exact amount of tax which the government was entitled to demand. I seem to recall that I cut short my visit in case he felt that there might have been some 'benefit in kind' had I overstayed my due time.

Thus, when the day of my visit to the local tax office dawned, I caught a bus – somehow it seemed appropriate, rather like taking one's hat off when going to church.

Most tax offices, for some unexplained reason, are situated on one of the higher floors of a multi-storied building invariably without a lift. Whether this is to deter visitors or to get them into such a physical state that they can be easily 'wound up' I cannot say. Perhaps it is so that their victims can be looked down upon. Having completed the long climb upstairs, I entered through a glass door, with 'HM INSPECTOR OF TAXES' stencilled ominously on the outside and 'OFFICE HOURS 10 A.M.-4 P.M.' written underneath. I pondered on this information. I knew I was venturing into Civil Service territory, but a six-hour day (do they eat?) seemed pretty laid back.

I entered a small room which had no floor covering and had a long serving counter divided into sections by partitions, presumably to give some impression of privacy. I saw a notice instructing me to ring a bell for attention, so I did.

Nothing happened immediately, but I imagined that a bell rang in some distant office, above which a notice might proclaim 'When this bell rings despatch junior (with sharpened pencil and notepad) to see what is happening', and so it was and a spotty-faced girl came out, holding a pad and pencil. It would seem that seventy per cent of callers had lost their way as at least two of the callers in my presence required the DHSS, one to claim some benefit, and the other to ask for the Job Centre. The DHSS was on the ground floor, but badly labelled. I can only assume that the DHSS was attempting to encourage their clients to take exercise.

I found it all rather depressing but stated my case as being that I wanted to clear up six years' arrears of tax muddle. The girl's eyes brightened. It was clear that she interpreted this as one might assess a murderer calling at a police station, and she disappeared without speaking to be replaced by a real inspector of taxes (he must have been all of twenty-three years of age). He looked disappointed when I explained that the Inland Revenue had all my returns for the past six years and that I wanted to know what they were doing about them.

Having taken my reference number, he returned to the anonymity of the inner office for a consultation, before returning with what I took to be a prepared statement aimed at convincing me that everything was being done in accordance with a prepared plan, rather like the military equivalent, 'retreating according to plan'. I swear that at this moment he had mounted a carefully placed footstool as he had apparently gained some three inches in height, and was looking down at me across the counter as he condescendingly said that 'they' would see me at 10 a.m. on the following Thursday. "In the private office," he added ominously. I mischievously asked if we might make it a Friday afternoon, knowing that tax inspectors like to be winding down their activities for the weekend by lunchtime on Friday. However the fledgling inspector looked so embarrassed that I felt I had scored a minor point, and I agreed that 10 a.m. Thursday would be possible.

I turned up promptly at 10 a.m. and went through the same procedure, except that the bright-eyed junior was expecting me and led me through a solid doorway into what I took to be the 'interrogation unit'. The room in which I found myself was about ten feet square and divided by a stout desk about four feet wide ('Too wide to jump over – significant,' I thought); this extended across the whole width of the room, and had two wooden chairs by it. The door closed and I imagined that the standing orders stated, 'Show taxpayer into room, and leave for 7 minutes', presumably to unnerve him. I do believe that Mrs Beeton might have written the standing orders!

After seven and a half minutes, the door on the opposite side of the desk opened and a pleasant woman entered ('Don't forget to smile at first meeting taxpayer') and sat down, carrying several thick files.

"Dr Ellis," she began, "your affairs are the most complex that have ever been seen in this office."

I responded, "Let's get one thing straight before we start. It's not my affairs that are complex, but rather your rules that are."

That seemed to get things started on the right foot, but then she started to quiz me on a number of matters. She enquired if I made up my own drugs. Not having even made up a prescription for over forty years, I jokingly explained that I was now off drugs, but she clearly didn't think that was funny. I even wondered if she thought I was a chemist. It was clear that she was fumbling in the dark and did not have the information which I had meticulously prepared and sent to her, and I said so.

She stopped and appeared to be searching the files which she had and considering what to do next. I was answering every question she put to me, and then suddenly she put the files down and said, "I might as well be frank as I don't believe you are trying to hide anything, and we really need your co-operation, for this reason: we have lost your files.

"*Lost* them?" I shouted, feeling that I was getting the better of the contest for the moment, and wishing to retain what I felt was a technical advantage.

She then went on to explain that some eighteen months ago they had had an intake of fresh staff, and by way of a training exercise they gave my files to a young trainee inspector with instructions that he must not do anything else till he had brought Dr Ellis's tax returns up to date. Months passed and this unhappy inspector-to-be became ill and started to take days off, claiming he was taking work home and he finally had a breakdown, clearly under stress.

At this juncture I felt a qualm of conscience as well as sorry for the inspector whom I was facing across the broad desk, but it did not last long I readily confess.

My inspector then explained that it eventually emerged that when the trainee inspector became ill (he had had a total breakdown and was eventually invalided out of the service), they asked for my files to be brought back to the office. Worse was to come, for under interrogation he confessed that one day, whilst in the habit of taking my files home, on the spur of the moment, whilst crossing the River Avon, he threw them all into the river. And so, with a most uncharacteristic Inland Revenue expression on her face, she said, "We now need your help to recreate your files."

I only half-believed her story, I felt I was on a 'true or false' panel game, but two events convinced me. The first concerned a subsequent episode in London, as told to me by a now-retired tax inspector. Apparently an overworked clerk in a tax office was taking tax papers home to catch up, and was increasingly under pressure, which was threatening his marriage. One evening, at Charing Cross station, which lies part way over the Thames, he impulsively threw some files out of the carriage window, and, as he thought, into the river. As luck would have it, a barge was passing by at the time, and the papers landed on its deck. The barge master, being an honest sort of man, found them, and returned them to the nearest tax office. History does not relate the rest of this story.

The second event occurred when, several years later, my tax affairs were transferred to another office ('tax district 15' – sounded like a prison block) and I went through a similar experience with a charming new six-feet, four-inches giant inspector of taxes. He gave the impression that he felt there was no need to cultivate the habit of 'looking down' at his prey; he just did it. He revealed that certain information was still missing from earlier years, unexplained in my files which had been transferred from the previous tax office.

"Strange," I heard him mutter, and he looked thoughtful.

After some time when the inspector searched again through the file, he looked embarrassed before saying, hesitantly, "I've been pondering about these 'gaps' in your returns... Have you... I mean... you weren't... sort of... well... 'out of circulation' for a while, by any chance?"

I felt sorry for him, especially looking around at his working conditions, when he suddenly apologised (unusual, I thought, for an official in the Inland Revenue), so I forgave him, hastening to explain about my previous tax district. He was visibly relieved and thereafter we had a most cordial relationship.

Before continuing he explained that they had to think along these lines, "As we do get some strange 'fast-track' visitors here."

Pausing at one page he suddenly chuckled, and explained that apparently some enthusiastic inspector had caused the tax machinery to send me a 'demand' for 6p, and apparently I had asked for a receipt, but there had been some light-hearted comments recorded in my file following the incident, evidence that there are some human beings behind the computer screens.

I am not sure whether the Inland Revenue have a form of confidential reports on their 'customers', but since then I am bound to say that in my dealings with them I have always found tax inspectors helpful and considerate, with the possible exception of the occasional officious junior on some minor matter.

I wonder if I've got some form of 'good conduct' mark on my file as they never seem to correspond with me any more, except for demanding payment!

Chapter Six
Stress

Stress is an enigma, and yet it is one of the most powerful factors to have a bearing on the destiny of the human race and, being for the most part self-created, *Homo sapiens* tenuously holds within his grasp the seeds of his own destruction.

Stress is now an integral part of modern daily living to a degree that has not yet been recognised as the threat it now is to our social fabric. Its effects are insidious, but germane to the purpose of this book and so have been given a section to themselves. Within that section, and under the general title of 'Stress', will be embraced a wide range of pertinent factors ranging from alcohol to suicide.

Though the word 'stress' is one of the more commonly used and misused words in the English language, most would claim to have had personal experience of it without comprehending the meaning or comprehension of the symptoms, results, or far-reaching effects of stress. It should therefore come as no surprise that the sequels go largely unrecognised.

Like pollution, the dangers to civilisation stemming from stress may not be recognised until it is too late to reverse the lemming-like rush to respond to the beckoning fingers of greed and self-interest.

Because of this widespread and significant influence that stress holds over both the human race as a whole and our lives as individuals it must have a bearing on the answer to the question, 'Why not live a little longer?'. It is for this reason that stress features at an early stage in this book, for much of the river of life and its quality stems from stress.

Stress is a natural ingredient in our daily lives and within normal limits would appear harmless enough; its presence is as inevitable as the waves in the ocean. Indeed, if absent, as on a dead calm sea, comment is called for: 'Isn't it quiet?' Don't be fooled, for if such apparent serenity were to continue for too long, paradoxically stress would appear in another guise – boredom:

> *Oh don't the days seem lank and long*
> *When all goes right and nothing goes wrong:*
> *And isn't your life extremely flat*
> *With nothing whatever to grumble at.*
>
> Gilbert & Sullivan, *Princess Ida*, Act III

Boredom as experienced on a long flight or long motor journey brings its own attendant dangers for the drivers – sleep.

A little stress, then, is not only beneficial but as essential as oxygen. An oyster without some 'stress' in the form of a irritant, when ingesting particles of sand during 'breathing', would not produce that beautiful end product, a pearl. In excess, both can become harmful, even, in the case of oxygen, poisonous, or, in the case of stress, harmful.

How much stress is necessary to keep a balance between boredom, and, at the other end of the spectrum, breakdown, will depend on circumstances.

Stress as a Management Tool

Skilful management will inevitably if unknowingly use stress to stimulate and inspire the management team. It might take the form of promoting a competitive spirit (hence the importance of 'games' in an adolescent's life), of inducements, constructive criticism (excess will cause 'strain' and be counter-productive), of working by example, and of good time-keeping. The degree of optimum stress will vary from individual to individual from time to time, as will the ease with which the stress can be surmounted.

When I was a small boy I was very shy, so much so that I dreaded going into a room full of people, and this persisted well into my teens. My embarrassment was obvious, so people would laugh at me, which didn't help matters one little bit, and in fact I would avoid meeting and mixing with people and became something of a loner. My father was exasperated, and one day pointed out that if I went into a room full of people I should remember that there would be at least one thing that I would be able to do better than anyone else in the room. Although I possibly never succeeded in finding out what that one thing was, it somehow gave me confidence, and when people started to laugh at me I started to laugh with them. Very gradually I discovered I could make people laugh and this has certainly helped to take the stress factor out of my own life.

My medical training taught me to enquire into what people do ('taking a medical history') in case there might be something in the patient's background which could explain the symptoms. This life-long habit is difficult to shake off so that I seem to find out without realising I'm doing it, what people's jobs are.

I suppose that I have made use of stress on occasions: for example, when I was chief executive of a sizeable organisation, I noticed that time-keeping amongst certain members of the regular staff was appalling, so I adopted the habit of occasionally and selectively leaving a handwritten message on the latecomer's desk requesting some information a.s.a.p. It worked wonders, and as a result I believe people respond to 'being wanted'.

So stress in moderation is beneficial, but how frequently modern living goes beyond what might be considered as acceptable must be increasingly brought into question.

How often does stress reach a level where tranquillity is upset? How does one recognise when this point has been reached? What can one do to combat it? What might happen if we do not take some remedial action?

Some anecdotes may illustrate these points. One thing is certain, a powerful antidote is to have a sense of humour, to laugh at oneself and at one's own stress-provoked predicament.

As modern living is full of stressful incidents, ample opportunity is provided to practise and develop these attributes. My own life has been filled with an abundance of potentially stress-provoking incidences, so I hope the reader will be able to share some of them and perhaps be reminded of similar incidents in his own life. By so doing he will be helped to assess what his 'stress tolerance' might be. Many stress-provoking experiences can even be humorous, though they may not immediately appear so to the victim, and hence the value of cultivating that sense of humour.

Stress can be and often is a significant factor in the undermining of health, even reducing life expectation and certainly the quality of life. If the quality of life falls below a certain, but unquantifiable level then the will to live is snuffed out, sometimes quite suddenly, thus swelling the suicide statistics. This can be seen in dire times as, for example, during serious economic disturbances such as in recessional times. Financial privation is a common cause of suicide, which tends to increase in such conditions. It is significant that the number of suicides is tending to increase, especially amongst young people.

Suicides: rank order of frequency (5,500 per annum – UK)

1) Pharmacists.
2) Dentists.
3) Farmers.
4) Medical practitioners (headed by psychiatrists).
5) Veterinary surgeons.

The common factor is that they all have access to poisons! What would the rest of us do if *we* had the same opportunity? As Dorothy Parker suggested:

> *Guns ain't lawful*
> *Nooses give;*
> *Gas smells awful;*
> *You might as well live*

Before we can discuss stress or even understand it as it affects our lives, a definition is called for. At once a difficulty arises, for there are two separate factors to be considered.

A) The first is the strict dictionary definition and for our purpose we need only look at that part of the definition which relates to humans. Here, *The Oxford English Dictionary* mentions three aspects:
   a) '...a demand on physical or mental energy' and 'the distress caused by this.'
   b) 'stressful – causing stress; mentally tiring...'
   c) In the context of physics, '...mechanical force per unit area exerted between contiguous bodies or parts of a body...'
   This now embraces physical torture such as corporal punishment.

B)   So that the medical consequences of stress might be considered, a simple additional definition is required: 'a problem which cannot immediately be resolved.'

A man was rowing on the Serpentine in Hyde Park, London, when he capsized. He came to the surface spluttering and waving his arms about wildly.

"Help – *HELP!*" he cried. "I can't swim!"

A passer-by shouted back to him, "Stand up, man, it's only four feet deep!"

Another problem solved, as many can be with a little thought or ingenuity.

The degree of stress is directly related to the significance of the problem. Missing a train might be no more than irritating (unless physically chasing it induces a fatal coronary); missing a flight could be more stressful; missing a diagnosis (or symptoms) might well be fatal in itself.

Stress is convoluted, for even fear of stress can prove stressful, such as when an actor 'dries'. Such fear or apprehension will bring on such a state of nervousness or anxiety accompanied by embarrassing symptoms such as perspiring, blushing (rare) or stuttering. There are many factors – the rarity of humility, abundance of aggressiveness, lack of general respect. I see it as a dangerous, insidious threat to mankind's future (i.e., the lack of it). If prolonged or repeated, this can lead to melancholia or hypochondria, possibly setting up a vicious circle of such intensity that medical advice has to be sought. In World War Two such a condition (not endorsed in medical circles) was called 'Lack of Moral Fibre' (LMF), which was the equivalent of 'shell-shock' in the earlier World War.

Everybody has a breaking point which will vary from person to person and according to circumstance, nature, and the level of the stress experienced. For some, it might be physical and for others social or even financial, of which the thirty-four suicides associated with the Lloyd's insurance market débâcle was a prime example. So what one person appears to be able to tolerate will bring about collapse in another, apparently brave and capable person.

The national pharmaceutical bill might provide a useful stress barometer and be an objective index of how the national 'feel-good factor' stands.

*

As a tendency to violence is one of the symptoms of stress, so the showing of violence on TV must be queried as a being a catalyst in the exercising of violence by those suffering from stress. Carried to a logical conclusion it might be argued that pharmaceutical companies have as much vested interest in the showing of violence on TV as have the tobacco companies in advertising the use of tobacco!

The human race is living today under the canopy of a battlefield, where a battle is being fought between Mother Nature and human scientists. As fast as man discovers an antidote, vaccine or 'wonder cure', Nature comes up with a new killer weapon. Within our own lifetime, the weapons deployed by nature have shifted from the 'infective' (neo-natal, scarlet fever, diphtheria, mastoid, pneumonia, tuberculosis, and many others caused by the bacteria family) to 'physical' diseases (diabetes, all cancers, coronary and other circulatory failures). The central nervous system 'parts failures' should also be included (Parkinson's disease, motor neurone disease, multiple sclerosis, Alzheimer's disease) and our 'own goal' should not be forgotten, self-induced smoking-related diseases, which account for at least 25% of all deaths.

During the last 15 years, however, nature has again reversed the weaponry back to 'infective' ailments, but this time has not been restricted to the 'tactical' bacterial weaponry, but has devised drug-resistant types, and has introduced a far more dangerous, strategic line of viruses, of which the AIDS virus is but a prototype; and so far neither a vaccine, nor a cure has been found. Such is the importance of this threat that a separate chapter is devoted to it, along with what other threats might be developed from this prototype killer strain.

One might have expected that as a group of illnesses was defeated so life expectancy would increase, but as fast as man has defeated a particular disease, nature has other killer diseases waiting to take their place, or has produced another variant of a previously contained one (TB is an example now reasserting itself once more). In this respect, mankind is assisting by scoring other 'own goals' apart from smoking, such as road traffic accidents, to give but one example.

If anyone has any doubt about nature's ability to develop and launch a new generation of weapons designed to eliminate the human race, they should read *The Common Plague* by Laurie Garrett, which makes AIDS seem about as threatening as the common cold!

Contrary to popular opinion, stress is not a direct killer, any more than the act of smoking a cigarette can terminate a life. In both cases, extended exposure to either can create conditions in which the body is weakened to such a degree that it becomes susceptible to an attack from a killer disease (in the case of smoking, cancer, heart attacks, etc.) which carries out the execution. Similarly, stress *per se* does not administer the *coup de grâce,* but so weakens the body's resistance and self-assurance that a further factor (often of an emotional nature) can precipitate a fatal incident, a heart attack or a stroke or a rupture of a main artery already weakened by other factors. This is why it is important to identify the sources of excess stress and remove them before permanent damage is done.

The Crush Syndrome

Modern living has become increasingly claustrophobic, not only as the result of physical overcrowding, but due to surveillance and intrusive routines, so that personal privacy is now at a premium, and, like the rats (see below), humans 'bite back' either vocally or by adopting threatening postures. This is most in evidence when exposure takes place in a public place or is exacerbated by exposure to the media, so that it can be witnessed on TV or by radio interviews, or, when Parliament is being televised, when the parties being exposed defend themselves by being aggressive to the point of rudeness and consequently become ineffectual. This is particularly in evidence at the Prime Minister's Question Time which has become a 'set piece' for cheap point-scoring rather than a useful opportunity for the dissemination of information. As such it might be compared to the stags' performance during the rutting season but with a less useful end product.

It is difficult to escape from the 'goldfish bowl society', and this provides an explanation of why personal cassette players have become popular, supplying a womb-like environment into which to retreat. Paradoxically, a blind man who is unable to 'observe' is much easier to talk to as a stranger than someone with normal 'observation antennae'.

Causes of Stress: Overcrowding

Experiments carried out with rats at the University of Pennsylvania demonstrated the effects of physical overcrowding.

A single rat was placed in a cage. After a few days it was showing evidence of boredom, relieved when a second rat was added. Then a third rat and a fourth and a fifth were added. All was well; even a fresh litter was born. Further rats were added until a number was reached at which the rats became quarrelsome, fighting over food, and eventually a degree of crowding was reached at which the irritability turned to fighting for no apparent reason and finally to cannibalism.

Other experiments with animals confirm that they stop breeding when their living conditions deteriorate, and they become irritable and quarrelsome under confined or crowded conditions.

In the case of the human race, the population explosion is only one of many factors contributing to overcrowding. Whether overpopulation is a euphemism for overcrowding or not, the effects show similarities to those seen in the overcrowded rats scenario.

Though at an early stage, dangerous and significant trends can be discerned developing in the human 'cage', as they were in the rat cage experiments. Though not identical – they are partially contained by the remnants of hundreds of years of 'civilisation conditioning' – they are none the less threatening to the continuance of life as we have come to know it.

We would ignore this trend at our and our children's peril. Cannibalism may have (only relatively recently though) been eradicated from human diets, but the existence of Dachau within our lifespan should remind us of what the human race is still capable of doing, should law and order irrevocably break down.

Robert Burns' 'man's inhumanity to man' could take on a new significance since he wrote 'Man was made to mourn' two hundred years ago.

As regards modern man's environment, 'overcrowding' has to be considered in a wider sphere than that of simple physical overcrowding when there are simply too many people in a static, designated area, although of course physical overcrowding in the extreme also has a devastating effect, as in ghettos.

'Packed like sardines in a tin' has become a cliché and of course represents the ultimate in overcrowding. Because there is no movement or body metabolism, no ill effects follow this particular type of overcrowding. But once movement is introduced, more space is required in direct proportion to the frequency, speed, distance and direction of movement.

The mental equivalent and achievement also contributes. 'Overcrowding', therefore, is influenced by many different circumstances; travel in any form exacerbates the consequences, whether it be frequency, speed, or even simply the converging of moving bodies.

Eliminate or reduce any one of these different factors and the problem is reduced proportionately, as for example by segregating vehicles on multi-lane roads. Railways take the solution a stage further by physically separating trains travelling in the same direction.

From time to time, however, the lessons are forgotten. In 1994, a fatal accident took place on the Uckfield branch railway line in Southern Britain when those in charge of policy decided to economise by removing the second track and permitting trains to travel on the remaining single line in opposite directions without any means of radio communication between them or with the signalmen to control them. Following the inevitable collision and at the subsequent enquiry, justification for the practice was given 'on the grounds of economy'!

Air travel takes the same principle of segregation one stage further by separating aircraft in a third, vertical plane. Even air travel has, however, reached saturation point, causing hold-ups around airports and spreading its own form of stress to those attempting to travel.

Speed also brings its own problems, especially on roads, even those within dual carriageways. Due to the inertia and varying reaction times from driver to driver, overcrowding of a different type causes multiple pile-ups between vehicles, even though they are travelling in the same direction.

The problem could be largely eliminated by the introduction of 'space segregation' measured, not by distance, but by a time interval between vehicles. For a relatively modest investment, drivers would be advised when they became too close (two seconds separation) to the vehicle ahead. 'Tailgating' accidents could be virtually eliminated, and the cost of the apparatus would pay for itself in less time than it takes to raise the index finger (the angry motorists' salute).

A two-second interval would be equal to a separation distance of some 40–50 metres at 60 m.p.h. (50–60 metres at 80 m.p.h.) between vehicles, and would eliminate the 'sheep-through-the-gate' syndrome so common on motorways today.

Under urban driving conditions the same time interval would enable vehicles to make more effective use of the limited road space by 'packing' together to within 20 metres per vehicle at 30 m.p.h.

A development of manual 'distance discipline' could be to control distance spacing electronically, whereby speed would be controlled automatically if the 'separation gap' was eroded, but subject to the driver being able to override for safety reasons. Variable speed limits have already been imposed on the more crowded section of the M25 motorway.

A bonus would be a better utilisation of police time, as control of speed by various manual devices would become as rare as checking railway train speeds, thus releasing police skills to be deployed on more productive tasks.

The 'speed kills' factor would be much reduced together with a welcome reduction of 'motorway madness' in the form of 'tailgating', not to be confused with the more modern and increasing phenomenon, 'road rage', which is stress-related whereas tailgating is pure ineptitude!

Though the population explosion and enhanced facilities for travel are the two main contributors to the stress factor, there are others, some related to these two, and others not so much. The effects of long distance travel, and jet lag are discussed elsewhere.

Environmental factors (pollution, poverty, living conditions) are all in their different ways contributing to stress, but are of a long-standing nature. Though overcrowding is a main source, isolation can also be, albeit rarely, a stress-provoking condition, just as noise is, especially when intermittent or variable in pitch. The body adapts even to relatively high noise levels in a remarkable way, just as it ignores the steady stream of stimuli bombarding you even as you read this sentence.

Here is a simple experiment:

Can you 'feel' the clothes you are wearing on your skin? Try a wriggle and, a pound to a penny I warrant you had not been aware of them till now!

A similar tolerance or ignoring of stimuli, is adopted in response to many other 'invasion of privacy' characteristics of modern living. These include 'junk mail' (straight into the bin?) the self-induced isolation of using a personal stereo or even of selecting an ex-directory phone number. A clubbing together into gangs reveals a need to belong rather than be exposed impersonally into modern life.

In spite of this, man is a sociable creature seeking contacts on a person-to-person basis. Such opportunities are increasingly rare in the work environment with the trend to large institutions, for example, cash dispensers replacing bank clerks, family solicitors being replaced by impersonal money-orientated 'faceless men', general practitioners dehumanised by practice managers, food shops replaced by supermarkets, and a trend towards a 'work-from-home' society.

Even the motor car has taken on an impersonal, detached personality, encouraging the driver to undergo a personality change which takes place when secluded in the motor car. It provides an environment in which the driver can dissociate himself from the unkindly, sometimes hostile, outside world, at which he can gesticulate aggressively from his secluded, seemingly detached eyrie! Feeling anonymously safe, he is encouraged to give vent to his road rage tantrums.

This aggression towards society is unwittingly encouraged by the example of police vehicles all too frequently travelling in 'full dress order' with wailing sirens, high-beam headlights, and flashing blue lights, inescapably adopting a very high profile, even an aggressive image, for other road users, and unwittingly encouraging imitation to a minority of, usually younger, attention-seeking drivers. Police bear a grave responsibility in deciding on the degree of urgency required when executing their onerous duties if the correct balance is to be reached between stealth and a state of full emergency and if the wrong example is not to be given, thus risking road rage assuming epidemic proportions, with the attendant accident risk.

In some European and African countries saturation point has been reached wherein ambulances as well as police vehicles never move without at least their flashing blue lights being illuminated; as a result everybody ignores them!

Even fear of stress can be stressful, inducing, for example, an anxiety neurosis, melancholia, or chronic hypochondria. Thus, although it is a very real condition, it can also be intangible.

Stress can be a major factor not only in health, but also in dying. Although the evidence is as yet scanty, the fact is now emerging that stress is not only psychological in its deployment, but also physiological, in that it would appear to interfere in some way with the body's autoimmune system. The Salisbury Common Cold Unit (Wiltshire), now closed, reported that many of their subjects under stress were twice as likely to catch a cold inoculated with the virus. It would not be unreasonable to expect that, in due course, research might offer evidence that a whole series of illnesses might be stress-related. Furthermore, as civilisation becomes more stressful, the whole pattern of diseases might be expected to alter, as indeed they are already doing. The result of this hypothesis might be the reduction of natural life expectation, depending on what sort of diseases are to flourish and, conversely, on what diseases are eliminated by scientific progress.

As stress is a major factor in the quest for longevity, how to avoid it, or the excess of it, and, if that can't be avoided, how to combat it, is important, and a number of stress-causing factors have been identified.

Though stress is not in itself a major killing factor it so weakens the body's strength that one can become susceptible to a number of lethal conditions, of which a coronary thrombosis is a common example.

Stress-causing events, together with a suggested score for each, are listed in Figure I. The list is not exhaustive but illustrates some of the more common stress-provoking factors. In themselves they may not be harmful, but if the victim has a family predisposition to coronary attacks they might be significant. The second point is that, although cumulative in the short term, relief from such events can over a few years return the 'risk clock' to zero again!

FIGURE I: STRESS FACTORS – PENALTY POINTS:

Score 200 units in any 3 years, and examine Coronary Risk Chart.

Persistent sex difficulties	39
Death of spouse	100
Divorce	73
Gain new family member	39
Marital separation	65
Marital reconciliation	47
Go to prison (variable)	63 (average may be from –25 to +125)
Marriage	50
Death of family member	39
Personal injury or illness	53
Loss of job	47
Retirement – age 45	45
Retirement – age 60	55
Retirement – age 73	20
Pregnancy (if married)	35
Pregnancy (if unmarried)	50
Business re-adjustment	39
Change in financial state	38
Change of work (same firm)	36
Change of work (different firm)	40
Wife stops work	26
Trouble with the boss (not wife)	23
Trouble with in-laws	29
Revision of personal routine	24
Extra-marital affair (start)	29
Extra-marital affair (finish)	20

FIGURE II: STRESS – CAUSE AND EFFECT

CAUSE	EFFECT
A. CROWDING • Living (cities) • Physical (housing) • Mental (persecution)	• Aggressive behaviour • Breakdown in human relationships
B. MOVEMENT • Frequency • Distance • Duration • Time Zones • Speed • Conditions	IRRITABILITY AND FATIGUE • Metabolic disturbance • Medical complications • Transitory confusion • Increased accident risk • Ditto, unless segregated • Modern travel 'erodes'
C. ENVIRONMENTAL • Temperature • Noise • Isolation • Poverty • General	ALL ABOVE PLUS: • Exhaustion • Intrusion of privacy
D. COMMUNICATIONS • Telephones • Fax • Mobile Paging	EROSION OF PRIVACY /RECUPERATION • Irritability • No time to consolidate event • Erosion of formative periods. Breakdown in conventions and manners
E. BUREAUCRATIC INTRUSIONS • At work • Personal • In public places (cars etc.) • At home ('cold canvassing')	'GOLDFISH BOWL' SOCIETY • Tendency to seek isolation or take refuge in groups/societies • Ditto • Personal stereos in public

F. HIGH PROFILE 'OFFICIALDOM' • Police (probing/aggression) • Security • Health papers (probing statistics)	THROUGH MIMICRY OF 'OFFICIALS' CREATES MIMICRY AND ROAD RAGE
G. Erosion of personal boundaries	A retreat into personal 'shell' or environment (clubs; personal stereos; ex-directory numbers)
H. Progressive erosion of 'honesty' by public officials; politicians.	Avoidance of responsibility – e.g., being 'economical with the truth'.
I. Absence of spiritual factor	Lack of conviction and self-confidence

CONCLUSION:
Over-familiarity leads to contempt. The slow but steady breakdown of social fabric and conventions leads to general medical complications, insomnia, alcoholism/drugs, circulatory problems, a coronary risk, acute and chronic depression and an increase in suicides. Related problems include marital breakdown, road traffic accidents, crime and (eventually) anarchy.

74

Effects of Stress (see Figure II)

How can stress affect health, well-being and the quality of life? When coexisting under conditions of ultra-close physical proximity, individuals of every species, especially human, need to have a private physical area available to which they can retreat from time to time, an area where one can be unobserved, rest and reflect or meditate according to the inclination of the moment. Intrusion into this area or the interruption of meditation even on a temporary 'visitation' basis can cause progressive stress, and will be resented and even resisted. This need for periodic solitude exists even at the height of a close 'mating' relationship and can be recognised in humans as well as in animals. Thus 'private time' is an essential ingredient for normal existence and prevention of stress.

Overcrowding as a cause of stress is not confined only to the physical, however. A private area also exists in the brain for 'reflective time', or mental digestion as it might be called. This covers periods when impressions and thoughts need to be collated and stored tidily in the appropriate memory bank if they are to be recalled efficiently at a later date. If these thoughts and reflections are not properly collated and filed at the appropriate moment they will become jumbled up or even forgotten for ever. Unless the brain is receptive to recording and storing in a rational manner for future reference, then experiences and conclusions will become muddled or even forgotten and, like any inadequate filing system, breakdown will surely follow with accompanying distress to those around.

Stress block. This is a condition which occurs when the brain becomes over-loaded and consequently 'freezes' or 'dries', to use theatrical language. Under these conditions not even a simple fact can be retrieved from the memory bank. The seriousness of the condition is not always recognised nor is it obvious to the casual onlooker, as the victim will devise a number of ruses to hide his predicament. It can be precipitated by a shock, and reported cases of memory loss, when somebody is found wandering aimlessly around, probably come into this category.

Recognition of such a state of affairs is important when rest is imperative, and it befalls to those around to recognise the seriousness of the condition before irreparable damage takes place. 'Rest sooner, rather than rest too late' should be the watchword; even in extreme cases, total rest should include detachment from the causal

FIGURE III: HYOTHETICAL CURVES RELATING PERFORMANCE TO ABILITY AND EXPERIENCE

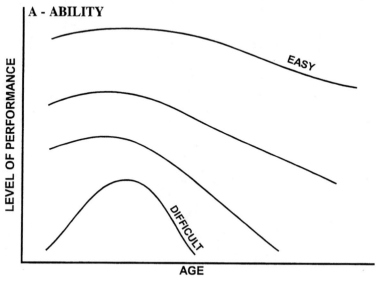

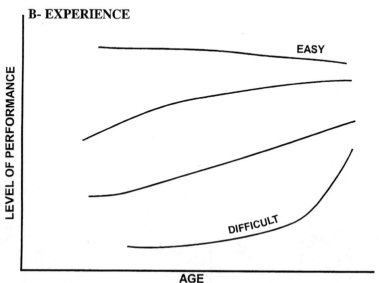

CONCLUSION: Experience is more important than ability, especially with difficult and stressful tasks.

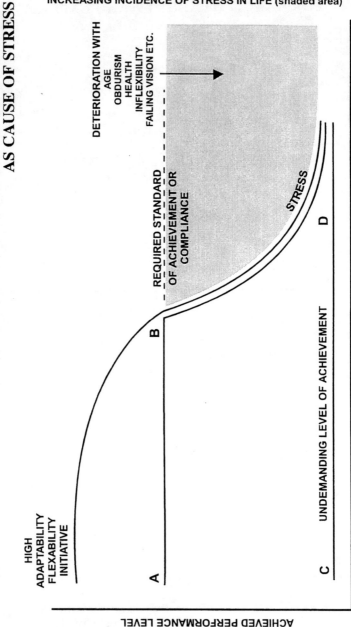

FIGURE IV: RELATIONSHIP BETWEEN DEMANDING PERFORMANCE AND AGE AS CAUSE OF STRESS

TREND FOR C - D LINE TO MOVE UPWARDS AND SO INCREASING INCIDENCE OF STRESS IN LIFE (shaded area)

HIGH
ADAPTABILITY
FLEXIBILITY
INITIATIVE

DETERIORATION WITH
AGE
OBDURISM
HEALTH
INFLEXIBILITY
FAILING VISION ETC.

REQUIRED STANDARD
OF ACHIEVEMENT OR
COMPLIANCE

A

B

STRESS

C

D

UNDEMANDING LEVEL OF ACHIEVEMENT

ACHIEVED PERFORMANCE LEVEL

AGE

HIGH STANDARDS OF ACHIEVEMENT DEMANDED (A - B) LEADS TO HIGH STRESS FACTOR
MODERATE STANDARDS OF ACHIEVEMENT DEMANDED (C - D) — BASES OF CONGENIAL LIFE

environment, albeit brief, to allow for a thorough medical examination to ascertain whether the breakdown is temporary or something more serious.

These passing references to extreme breakdown should not be thought of as alarmist, for we all live in these modern times, from crisis to crisis, but, like a ship at sea rising to the swell, we surmount the daily pressures as they arise and without too much disturbance to our overall efficiency. Without a modicum of stimulation, life would be dull. However that ultimate breaking point following exposure to excess stress is often nearer than might be apparent to friends or work colleagues, especially if the victim has a 'high threshold'. It is important to remember that every person has an ultimate breaking point and if pressed too far this will be breached.

Different persons have varying susceptibilities to different forms of stress. The dangers, for example, of pushing the mind and body when exposed to significant time zone variations is commented on, and at such times the tolerance to other forms of stress is markedly lowered. This particular form of stress did not exist before the age of jet travel when a return trip by sea at leisure ensured that recreation and reflection was taken.

Communication is another source of stress, for the telephone carries priority. How often does one find oneself indulging in serious discourse in an office or in a shop or at home whilst entertaining, when the phone rings and the caller brashly, if innocently intrudes into one's privacy? Here is an example of how 'manners' (which are simply a form of 'anti-stress') need updating, and it would be therapeutic if all phone calls were prefaced by a question: 'Is it convenient?'

Privacy is at a premium, for the advent of the mobile telephone has marked a major erosion of personal privacy. A code of conduct is required for the use of mobile phones in public places, especially in public conveyances. Can you be sure that your movements are not being recorded on some unseen closed-circuit television camera?

Politicians and other public figures are the most exposed, and their facile replies to public questioning by the media underpin the lack of regard for them. They reduce performance to an almost meaningless level, for fear of self-incrimination, and encourage a policy of 'being economical with the truth'.

'Junk mail' is yet another example of an intrusion into privacy, as are cold canvassing sales techniques, of which telephoning must surely be the worst.

Trials and tribulations beset any public, and especially political figures today, resulting from technological 'advances' in the field of communications. These erode everybody's personal privacy and constitute yet another form of overcrowding, thus accentuating stress. Simultaneously, standards of honesty are reduced by encouraging deviousness rather than enhancing open-handedness.

Not all situations causing stress are serious and they can be amusing, even hilarious, except to the one at the centre. One such scene concerned myself. Perhaps it should be recorded that I seem to have a propensity for getting into embarrassing situations, and my only consolation is that it seems all too frequently to cause merriment to others.

I was attending a rather 'splendid' dinner party, where I knew one had to be on one's best behaviour, and consequently felt rather nervous. Anticipating grace, I had remained standing by my chair, and was put at ease when my host proclaimed, somewhat tersely, I thought, "We haven't got a padre with us – thank God," and sat down.

I found myself placed next to a rather frumpy woman, dressed in a long dress, matching the equally long linen table cloth, which overhung the table almost down to the floor. Having helped my dinner companion into her seat, I endeavoured to pull myself into the table, but was frustrated by what seemed to be a forest of table legs.

Not wishing to be left out of the party, I finally pushed my legs as far as I could under the table, at the same time lifting the table cloth up to allow my knees entry.

In one of those moments when that inevitable silence falls on the gathering, my companion, with a morsel of food delicately balanced on her fork, halfway to her mouth, paused in mid-bite, so to speak, and in an unnecessarily loud voice, turned to me, and said, "Do you mind, Doctor, you've already got my skirt nearly up to my navel, and I'm not too sure what is going to happen next."

Stress is insidious in the way it infuses its damaging influence into our lives. The evidence is all around us, although not always recognised. The growing breakdown in marriages is often attributed to a lowering of 'standards', be they religious, moral, or concerning promiscuity or materialism, but mistakenly stress is put down as a sequel rather than a cause when it is both. We are increasingly living in a scrambled-egg society where everything is muddled up and guidelines and standards have become obscured.

Smoking and Alcohol:

Both of these factors affect health in a general sense. They also both neatly feature in a discussion on stress as they can both be revealing as symptoms.

Smoking features elsewhere as a major cause, not only of illness, but also of premature death. Alcohol also can, when taken to excess, contribute to injuries and death, as in road traffic accidents (RTAs).

Alcohol

Alcohol is a sedative and is resorted to frequently under conditions of stress. It is also recognised that alcohol has many social benefits (and dangers) and, as such, plays a major part in society.

Alcoholism as an addiction can play a significant part in mental and physical illness as well as in premature death; specifically, alcohol's role in the causation of RTAs is relevant, and will be discussed later.

How Much Alcohol is Safe?

It has been suggested that the safe upper limit for regular alcohol intake is 21 units a week for a male, and 14 units for a female. In round figures, one unit can be considered as half a pint of beer or a single measure of spirits. This figure was arrived at as being the 'all round' upper safety level for virtually everybody, but clearly this is the philosophy of the 'convoy rule' (i.e., the speed of a convoy is that of the slowest ship). Real life is different, for we are of different weights, shapes, fat content, etc. For example, a different figure is given for males and females, for the simple reason that, on average, females are lighter in weight, and also because they have more body fat than males; fat, having a poor blood supply, does not absorb alcohol to the same degree as other tissues. This means that the rest of the female body, including various organs (liver etc.)

absorbs more alcohol than in an equivalent male, and therefore, unit for unit, is more susceptible to damage.

Many factors will influence whether a person might be damaged by imbibing alcohol regularly over an extended period. These factors include weight, general state of health, medical history, susceptibility to alcohol, ability to metabolise it, tolerance, consistency of intake, and also age.

For views on the beneficial effects of alcohol, I would refer to the findings of the Common Cold Unit at Salisbury, now closed, where it was discovered that a modest amount of alcohol could give some protection against the common cold. This may be coupled with other findings that a modest daily alcohol intake actually increases one's life expectancy.

I was finally convinced by the published thoughts of Sir Richard Doll who, with Sir Bradford Hill, first discovered the relationship between smoking and lung cancer. He also convincingly demonstrated the beneficial effects of mild to moderate alcohol consumption on diminishing the risk of dying from heart disease.

In 1995, a team from the Department of Public Health at West Glamorgan Health Authority went further, and it is worth reporting their findings at length for the benefit of those who might have taken fright at the earlier reports of maximum safety being 21 (male) or 14 (female) units per week. The Glamorgan lot, however, are far more reassuring!

They categorised weekly alcohol consumption as follows:

Category	Classification	Units per week (Female equivalent)
A	Non-drinkers	Nil
B	Mild drinkers	21 (14)
C	Moderate drinkers	21–49 (15–34)
D	Severe drinkers	Over 49 (34)

Of the 827 participants:

40% were non-drinkers (category A)
49% were mild drinkers (category B)
85% were moderate drinkers (category C)
25% were severe drinkers (category D)

Put another way, I read this as 'permitting' 3 large spirits per day, but anybody reading this must make up their own mind as regards their own inclination and habits.

The report went on to observe that the 'mild to moderate' drinkers enjoyed 'significantly better health experience' than did the non-drinkers; they 'perceived themselves to be more physically active... experienced less bodily pain, more vitality and were generally more sociable than the non-drinkers'.

The report concluded that 'mild to moderate alcohol consumption seems to confer not only longevity but also a better quality of life related to health'. The apocryphal story of the apostle Paul advising Timothy 'to take a little less water and little more wine' appears to be scientifically sound and valid.

Alcohol and Driving

As with smoking, although the supporting statistics are clear, the interpretation of those statistics, and remedial measures which should be taken, have been clouded by emotional overtones. This is understandable, for injuries and deaths do generate emotions of a substantial level. The purpose of this section is to see where there is common ground in the objective.

Objective: To reduce road traffic accidents, minimise injuries, and if possible eliminate deaths.

There can be no justification for the condoning of driving whilst being impaired to any degree by alcohol. Alcohol still remains a major causal factor in vehicle accidents, and the campaign against this scourge over the past twenty years has been fully justified.

1982: 42,265 drivers were breathalysed; of whom 29.3% tested positive. There were 1550 alcohol-related deaths from accidents in 1982, 15% of all road deaths being pedestrians. However, the number of pedestrians *and* those who had consumed alcohol was not published, so it is suspected that there could probably have been an element of 'double counting' included in this 15% figure – an important consideration, as inebriated pedestrians can be a factor in alcohol-related accidents on the road – including deaths – and this would distort the 'alcohol at the wheel' figures.

1993:The breathalyser failure rate had fallen dramatically to 6.6%, having been 29.3% ten years earlier, and alcohol-related deaths had fallen to 550, pedestrians still included. Provisional figures for 1994: 510. Clearly the right targets (other than pedestrians) were being identified.

The Hard Core

There still remains a much reduced and relatively small number of drivers who drink and drive and are responsible for the now relatively small number of alcohol-related accidents.

Who are they, and how can they be identified and then eliminated?

Figures relating to 1994 reveal three significant facts:

a) More than half the drivers killed or seriously injured in road accidents are aged 25 or younger.

b) The highest group of drivers failing breathalyser tests are aged between 20–24, and significantly...

c) 16% of all licensed drivers are in the 17–25 age bracket and this group is responsible for 52% of all road deaths and serious road injuries.

The policies, however, have not been changed in the light of this success, and, as wringing out a wet towel has its limitations in extracting moisture, there is now a case for reviewing the policy in order to continue achieving success without eroding public goodwill by harassing innocent drivers unnecessarily.

Christmas 1994: During the twelve-day Christmas period, 78,090 breath tests were carried out (for all reasons), of which 4,720 (6.04%) were positive. Throughout the whole of 1994, 680,000 tests were carried out; of these 14% were positive. It was estimated that 1 in 5 drivers killed in this period were over the legal limit, compared to 1 in 4 in 1984.

In Sussex, a county renowned for its fierceness regarding offences relating to alcohol, a series of 'random checks' on vehicles were carried out over a two-day Christmas period in 1994: 2716 vehicles were stopped at road blocks, and 131 drivers were breathalysed (4.8%), but only one (0.037%) was successfully prosecuted. Thus, 2716 drivers were stopped at random, ostensibly for an 'unstated' reason, without causing any apparent danger or accident to anyone, to achieve one prosecution.

Christmas 1995: The levelling out in positive breathalyser tests seen in the previous two years continued, and appears to have stabilised at around 6%. This hard core of offenders is concentrated in the 30–45-year-old age bracket.

If further progress is to be made towards the elimination of alcohol-related accidents a change of policy is called for, one which should not alienate the remaining considerable public goodwill towards the police in their difficult task.

The Way Ahead

If the hard core of drivers who are the cause of alcohol-related accidents are to be targeted, there needs to be a revision of policy:

a)   Legal limit: this is inadequate, for at the present legal limit the chances of being involved in an accident are already doubled.

b)   The present obligatory forfeiture of the driving licence for a mandatory period of at least 12 months is a blunt instrument and is no longer as effective in achieving the objective:

   • It takes no account of whether there has been impairment due to alcohol that has caused damage or even inconvenience to others.

   • It undermines the discretion of the bench, a fundamental cornerstone of the magisterial system.

   • It fails to catch those who are below the legal limit whose driving may still be impaired by alcohol.

   • It is indiscriminatory in its punishment, destroying some and letting others off without even inconvenience.

   • It is imprecise in that, unlike exceeding a speed limit, it penalises the ultra cautious and encourages the 'abandoned' person to take a chance, the very person who is of an irresponsible inclination.

   • It is largely unselective, in that, with 'random testing' (in all but name) the safe driver is tested along with the unsafe.

The 'Zero' Alcohol Option

This would have the following advantages:

i) It would uncover the driver who was already at twice the risk (see (a.) above).

ii) It would restrict breathalysing to:

- Anyone involved in an accident.

- Anyone committing a moving traffic offence

- Anyone driving in a grossly erratic fashion or indulging in 'attention seeking' behaviour.

One could also introduce a new offence, either in addition to the present one, or preferably after a trial period along the following lines: anybody found to have any detectable alcohol in their body (or a specified minimum – to avoid 'rogue' readings) shall be guilty of an additional offence, having been found guilty of (ii.) above. Being a less serious offence, a commensurate penalty should apply.

Advantages:

- It would introduce an element of self-judgement, in that, if one has taken any alcohol at all, very great care would be taken, and this in itself should result in a marked reduction of the accident rate.

- It would be economical in terms of police manpower, releasing patrols to concentrate on non-alcohol-related offences which are themselves a major cause of remaining accidents.

- It would foster better relations between law-abiding motorists and the police, in that motorists would not be stopped without purpose.

- It would reinforce the proper objective, i.e., the elimination of accidents rather than the elimination of alcohol, and encourage sober and responsible social behaviour.

The number of deaths from road accidents has now been overtaken by suicides. They both have a common thread of self-destruction. However, serious injuries are at eight times the number of deaths – this should not be forgotten in all the above considerations.

The Alternative?

Failure to target the alcoholic hard core of this problem, and indiscriminate breathalysing, will materially change the social habits and fabric of the community. The objective should be the elimination of accidents, not the elimination of alcohol, except where the latter is the cause of the former. The alternative is to risk that the 'baby' (paradoxically, the older driver) is thrown out with the 'bathwater' (younger middle-aged driver).

Meanwhile we are left to survive as best we can under the present regime which includes 'random testing' in all but name.

*

The Spiritual Factor

This has deliberately been left until last, not because it is not important, for it may well be the most important factor of all, but because it has ethereal qualities which to some are difficult to grasp. Although some may take the view that it is lacking in substance, the spiritual factor is probably the one single factor with the strength to hold society together and halt its apparent slide towards extinction.

How might this be brought to bear? Somehow an understanding common to all religions should be sought, and this might be founded on two pillars:

i)   A reference book: this does not have to be the same book for everybody. It would assume that common standards can be found in every religion's Bible or book.

ii)   Tutors (priests) who are available to guide and interpret everybody's needs. In spite of the self-agonising period which the Church as a whole is going through, priests as individuals generally command a respect which may well be the envy of other professional people.

What better challenge than for the Church to give a new lead to society by calling for a reappraisal of circumstances and updating its own teachings to match present-day problems. Current standards are now too deeply established to reverse, and the Church should adopt them rather than continuing to 'command' a return to bygone standards, as turning the clock back is no longer regarded as being a practical option.

It would entail embracing many modifications to the interpretation of what is right or acceptable, or even practical. Perhaps a new tolerance, even acceptance towards divorce could be a good starting point?

Regrettably, I feel unable to take the subject much further, for I do not feel sufficiently well-qualified to do so, but I do feel a need as I believe many others do.

Conclusion

Stress has now reached endemic proportions in First World countries and should be considered to have assumed national characteristics as well as affecting individuals. As such, nations might well be classified in accordance with their 'stress-provoking lifestyles', measured possibly by a 'basket' of characteristics and statistics including such variables as homicide and suicide rates, divorce rate, incidence of mental illness, unemployment, house repossessions and many others. The whole could be fed into, and possibly set against the gross national product, before arriving at a 'national-feel-good' factor or a realistic 'standard of living'. It might well reveal a new list of 'desirable' countries in which to reside.

Chapter Seven
Argentosis

I am a millionaire: That is my religion.

George Bernard Shaw

The love of money is the root of all evil.

1st Epistle of Paul to Timothy 6:10

Strictly speaking, argentosis is more a syndrome than a disease, but because its effects are both insidious in onset, far-reaching in effect, and devastating in result, it is perhaps more appropriate to consider it as a disease. As yet, it has not been identified by name; I propose that this omission now be rectified.

Origin

Plato used to tell his pupil, Aristotle, that within a community no one person should earn more than five times the wage of the average worker. Within broad limits that rule of thumb had not been grossly breached (allowing for changes in living standards and technological advancement) until modern times, indeed until after World War II. Historically, America has always led the 'inequality' ratio. By 1969 Plato's ratio had widened in the US to 7.5, and by 1992 to 11, followed by Australia (9.7), New Zealand (8.6) and Switzerland (8.5). Japan and Germany were the most equal (around 5), with Britain just over 6, though there is evidence of a rapidly widening occurrence in Britain since 1992. In 1995, the early evidence would indicate that Plato's ratio has reached a differential of 12, which is not sustainable.

The effect of a widening, or already widened ratio between rich and poor leads to many problems of a divisive and consequently stressful nature. Any situation where high differentials exist, whether it be meteorological (storms), electrical voltage (shocks), high blood pressure (strokes etc.) or just plain envy, all lead to trouble, and it is within that context that 'argentosis' has a place in this book. (Further reading can be followed in *The Bell Curve* by psychologist Richard Herrnstein, and in *Paying For Inequality* from the Institute for Public Policy Research.)

Like many diseases, for example tuberculosis, evidence can be found as far back as Biblical times of the pre-existence of argentosis, although it was not the scourge that it has become in modern times. Silver was designated as a bargaining entity, and in the New Testament St Matthew suggested that man might be traded for thirty pieces of silver.

Other than the occasional miser, the incidence of 'money poisoning' was minimal through the Middle Ages, and has only reached epidemic proportions since World War II. Catalytic conditions for its spread can probably be laid at the doors of the accountancy profession, accompanied by the wider effects of overpopulation and consequent overcrowding, linked to the explosion of information technology encouraged by inflation.

Accountants invented the cult of the effective use of money, putting it to work rather than letting it lie idle. This, in turn, turned the focus on a similar effective use of goods and time in business, so that anything which was lying idle had to be banished or put to a money-producing role. It is now extended to human beings.

This in its turn, stood values on their heads, coining the phrase of money-oriented people who 'knew the price of everything but the value of nothing'. I recall a service department of a very large motor dealer in Leeds which had installed a coffee-vending machine on the service counter. The company accountant, in his zeal, apportioned every square foot a part of the overheads of the whole company, including those occupied by the coffee machine. Viewed thus, the price per cup of coffee had to be trebled in order to show a commensurate profit. The machine fell into disuse and thus was dispensed with, causing many dissatisfied customers to take their custom elsewhere!

One of the symptoms of argentosis is greed, and when fully developed, the victim's whole character undergoes a change as the seeking of money has sublimated virtually all else to a secondary and low priority role. In the pursuit of this mythical substance, truth has given way to half-truths, if not to lying. Personalities change, and such is the power and even addiction, that families are destroyed due to a neglect of anything of substance except money. Self-respect becomes confused and, providing the victim can escape detection, dishonesty becomes a ready tool. The better human characteristics disappear through lack of use so that manners and courtesy become superficial shams. Even work targets become obsolete unless money-orientated. Eventually society destroys itself, as the only end product becomes money: an end in itself rather than a means to an end. Thus, in the end, money ceases to be beneficial, and becomes a poison, destroying everything in its path including its host just as any cancer does.

The cure? This is easy to prescribe but difficult to take. The answer, perhaps surprisingly, does not lie in egalitarianism, for no two people have identical needs. Moreover there are different needs for capital and income. The healthy man without a family may be able to meet his personal needs with very little capital but a moderate income as his hobby might be helping the disadvantaged, whereas the family man with many children beginning to earn their living might require some capital to provide a roof, but little income. Another, disabled, but with a long life expectation, may need both income and capital. In short, it is difficult to justify the enormous sums of money changing hands. These are at present out of all proportion to anybody's actual or potential needs.

The Americans tend to have natural immunity to argentosis. As a nation they respect it, pursuing the earning of money with vigour, but, once earned, they tend not to hoard it, neither nationally nor as individuals, but are generous to less fortunate nations, causes and individuals alike. This attitude appears to confer a degree of natural immunity to the ravages of the syndrome itself.

This immunity is enhanced by the national attitude towards large differentials between the rich and the poor. 37% of Americans said yes when asked if large differentials were necessary for economic growth, compared with 25% of Britons, 23% of Germans and 9% of Dutch.

Turning to argentosis as a disease, rather than a syndrome, how would it be described in a textbook of medicine? Probably under the section headed 'Psychological Medicine'. It might read like this:

Psychiatric disorders associated with Social Maladjustment: the Argentosis Syndrome.

The varieties of form and course of the organic psychiatric disorders associated with money are still fortunately relatively few, although there are several indications that they are on the increase. There is a grave danger that they may well undermine the whole structure of society in much the same way that a flock of sheep can damage one another should they all strive to get through a gate together. A parallel to sheep may be seen in humans when closeted in motor vehicles on crowded highways, when otherwise conventional manners are subjugated or overridden.

Similar symptoms in a minor degree can be observed in the animal kingdom, as, for example, in squirrels collecting an excess of nuts or even the domestic dog hiding a bone. No practical advantage is to be gained by this irrational act, for, although great pretences of secrecy are demonstrated during the burying, considerable difficulty appears to be encountered during the retrieval, and a thankful return to the bowl labelled 'DOG' soon ensues. Magpies also show a form of early argentosis. Susceptibility for succumbing to argentosis is difficult to predict, though it can be understandable in relation to the patient's previous experience in life; hence a careful history is essential when drawing up a prognosis.

The syndrome, and the associated symptoms, should be described before investigating how different personalities and circumstances might succumb or be immune when exposed to the temptation.

The syndrome can be compared with leukaemia (cancer of the white blood corpuscles) in that the corpuscles, like money, are essential for living. However, in the case of leukaemia, if the white cells start to increase significantly, they take over and strangle the whole blood circulatory system, replacing it with the cancerous white cells. Eventually the normal physiological function of the blood and vital organs (which depend on an adequate blood flow to supply them with life-bearing oxygen) ceases, and death ensues. As the illness progresses, the patient's whole physical character changes, and he or she looks ill and is unable to lead a normal life; in the case of leukaemia, periodic blood transfusions prolong life and bring temporary relief. In the case of argentosis, however, the reverse is the case; draining off the excess funds comparable to the now disused practice of 'blood-letting' for high blood pressure, may give some relief by depriving the victim of the source of his compulsion, although relapses are likely.

Definition

An obsessive preoccupation with the accumulation of money or money derivatives such as shares on options.

Method

Excessive charging for services rendered, seeking to render services unnecessarily, or exaggerating such services in the pursuit of inward cash flow, the whole being defended by quoting 'official' rates for the task; solicitors are particularly prone to this.

Synonyms

Greedy; rapacious; obsessional; gold-digger (usually applied to females).

Pathology

No overt pathology is evident in the early stages of the syndrome, though a propensity for 'creature comforts' develops in the later stages, and any tendency towards alcoholism must be guarded against.

Incidence

Either sex may be affected, though the morbidity is predominantly male-orientated due to the male's greater exposure to the causal environment. The male sufferer is known as an argentote. In the female (an argentottie), the symptoms are more covert and the results more devastating and debilitating to third-party victims; this leads to a high stress incidence in any male who might come into contact with an argentottie. Argentotties employ a wide variety of equipment, most of it very basic, to capture their quarry, but, like fishermen's flies, their bait is reusable, and is not always brought into play. Ancillary ploys are sometimes used instead, which often attracts the interest of the tabloid press. This can lead to complications such as notoriety, which can further the argentottie's cause if played skilfully. When this occurs the only effective treatment is to move the patient's victim into an isolated environment, until matters settle down; during this phase, bank balances need careful monitoring in case an ensuing haemorrhage requires a financial transfusion (or even a tourniquet in the case of extreme financial loss).

In uncomplicated cases of argentosis, the male sufferer is more common, and his presence is easily spotted, especially in high-density business areas. The widespread use of, and dependence on computers has encouraged the criminal argentote in the pursuit of his goal. There is now less tendency for individual financial transactions to be perused, as was the case pre-computer, when humble clerks with or without a quill pen would double check bookkeeping entries and in turn be checked themselves. Implicit trust in the computer has widened the scope to divert cash into mythical accounts without being questioned.

Age

Tends to affect middle- and later-aged males, often deserted by their family unless the spoils are temptingly displayed. Lawyers are particularly prone to the condition ('ambulance chasing' should be regarded with suspicion); other lawyers may be sighted grazing in the company of argentosis victims, offering advice for which fees are rendered.

Signs and Symptoms

Tendency to obesity (through 'good living'), paying undue attention to financial publications such as the *Financial Times*, *Investor's Chronicle* and similar papers. Other symptoms include:

The seeking of personal contracts for directors of large industrial companies, preferably quoted or newly privatised, an appetite for 'roll-over' service agreements with suitably lucrative termination clauses, and attached share options, all of which are pathogenic.

Ex-government ministers are particularly susceptible, and need isolating during the quarantine period.

Other telling signs include a propensity for a variety of perks, such as attractive insurance, including health, and insurance covering extreme, but not unknown events, such as death from suicide; a preoccupation with visible status symbols, including lavish forms of personal transportation; admission to well-publicised (and well-media-covered) public entertainment events, such as sports, racing, the arts etc.

Predisposing Causes

Extreme poverty, frustration of a career due to poverty, unhappy marital circumstances, heavy debt, inadequate personality or substandard physique have been known to precipitate a compensatory need to amass wealth. Even an inability to read and write can fortuitously bring on a lesser, but rewarding, version of the syndrome.

Course and Progress

The syndrome tends to be habit-forming. It is usually progressive and resembles many physical malignancies in that it tends to consume the personalities of victims, who can be perceived to have undergone a personality change; once generous, they tend to become self-seeking. An associated manifestation is power-seeking by self-aggrandisement; seeking recognition through spurious titles appears when the lack of real life success becomes apparent. Ironically, these very titles have a tendency to lose their impact as their owners advance in years and are assessed for their intrinsic self-worth, rather than their trappings. These 'social trinkets' lose value as the number of holders increases.

The prognosis is grave when material possessions, and particularly the accumulation of money, becomes an end in itself rather than a means to an end.

Complications

Marital breakdown, alcoholism, a variety of mental illnesses, legal problems, even crime as the syndrome spurs one on towards an imagined goal. Friends and respect become elusive, thus aggravating the condition.

Prognosis

Probably some reduction in life expectancy, alleviated by an ability to provide adequate creature comforts; ultimate loneliness and oblivion, frequently in a foreign country in an effort to avoid inheritance tax, which is often thwarted by a final return to the mother country to seek medical treatment for a terminal condition.

Treatment

Like alcohol, total abstinence, and insulation from the cause, possibly by denying all wealth (trusts etc.); taking holy orders, or taking up residence in a monastery have both been known to be beneficial.

Prophylaxis

No vaccine known, but the syndrome is less prevalent, or at least less contagious, in times of war, and ironically thrives under conditions of excess. Under conditions of shortage, the motivation is to replace that shortage by creation, which can have a beneficial effect on society.

> *All progress is based on a universal desire...*
> *to live beyond one's means*
>
> Samuel Butler (1612–1680)

So perhaps the price of progress is greed, which, in an attenuated form, could form the basis of an argentosis vaccine!

Lloyd's (of London) and greed have been cited as an illustrative factor in this syndrome. The Lloyd's débâcle of 1988–92 has been, along with a number of pension failures, possibly the largest single series of personal financial failures in the history of capitalism, certainly since the 'South Sea Bubble' in 1720. It has caused individual and family breakdowns on an unprecedented scale, including many bankruptcies, untold family breakdowns, several suicides, and at least 16,000 families have been severely damaged financially, either directly or indirectly, on a scale hitherto not believed possible. It has also led to the largest collective series of civil actions ever to be brought to the English courts.

The underlying cause of argentosis on a global scale is greed on an unprecedented scale. However, contrary to public opinion, the greed and argentosis lay not with the 'outside' names at Lloyd's – 'sheep waiting to be sheared' as Robert Hiscox, one time Deputy Chairman of Lloyd's referred to them – but with the working members of Lloyd's. Large numbers of these 'inside' names became argentotes, and argentotties, with the consequent destruction of any sense of propriety or guilt, although there were a few exceptions who had a natural immunity to the syndrome. The predominant presenting symptom displayed by these 'shepherds' – the professional 'inside' names controlling the Lloyd's market – was arrogance, together with greed for themselves, leading to many of their downfalls, and in so doing, ruining many of the 'outside' names in the process. They were obsessed with the myth of their own competence coupled with a belief that they would not be found out.

Within the square mile of the city of London, argentosis reached epidemic proportions on a scale that could only be compared with that of myxomatosis in the rabbit population. It is to be hoped that a form of auto-immunity will evolve, though whether the removing of the privilege of 'self-regulation' from Lloyd's will inevitably and justifiably be the price to be paid raises some doubts.

This chapter would not be complete without a brief reference to the fact that a deficiency of money can be just as destructive at the other end of the scale to argentosis. As in many medical diseases the effects can be devastating when measured on the social scale. Just as a deficiency in dietary intake leads to illness, such as an inadequate level of vitamin C can lead to scurvy, or of vitamin B to beriberi, so a shortage of money can lead to crime but of a different, more opportunistic type to that caused by excess. As in any shortage, the remedy lies in replacement therapy, by the provision of money or the essentials which money can buy, but it is important to start the treatment before irreversible personality changes have set in, or, for that matter, health deterioration, which can even lead to a terminal result.

> *You know what God thinks of money*
> *when you see to whom he gives it*
>
> Anon

Chapter Eight
Circadian Rhythm

The Body Clock

As already explained, this book is not intended to be a medical textbook, so there is no need to be alarmed by the main title. The phrase 'body clock' is the key, even though the body clock is a poor timekeeper, always running slow.

This was discovered in the 1950s by isolating a group of people, and divorcing them from all forms of timely contact with the outside world. This was achieved by placing the subjects in a 'sealed environmental unit' with no windows, so that it was not possible for them to have reference to the sun, and therefore they were unable to say whether it was day or night; there were no clocks or other references to time, actual or elapsed.

They were left for several weeks, but their brief was to live as normal a day-to-day life as they could manage from what their bodies were telling them, to keep to daily routines like going to bed, sleeping, eating, getting up, and generally to adopt a routine similar to their normal habits, guided entirely by what their body clocks told them.

They were asked to keep a diary, and estimate how many days had passed. They were to estimate when they thought they had been isolated for 24 days (to make a numerical resemblance to a 24-hour day). On finishing their experiment, the subjects were astonished to find that, whereas they believed they had passed 24 days, in fact 25 days had passed! They had lost a day in their biological lives for ever. It was as though they had crossed the International Date Line.

With advancing years, the body clock runs even slower, giving its owner the impression that real time is flying by – similar to a slowing train being overtaken by a passing express.

There is insufficient data to conclude that, by throwing away our timepieces and relying solely on our bodily clocks, we would extend our natural lives by one year every 24 years. However it might just be possible that, left to its own pace of progression, there might be a little less stress on the bodily systems. It's a theory not to be recommended though, as making appointments with other earthly mortals might become difficult, especially if your daytime coincided with someone else's night-time. This could be rather like being on 'moon-time', as one subject suggested, a little later each day. Perhaps we were designed to live on the moon, and some quirk of fate has placed us on the wrong planet!

The body clock has another characteristic. Unlike chronometers, it has an varying strength of 'tick', beating more strongly by day than by night. The strength of the tick is called the metabolic rate, similar to a domestic furnace which provides hot water. It 'burns' at a higher rate at certain times of the 24-hour cycle than at others. It is remarkably consistent and can only be altered over a period of some days by a variation in the daily life pattern. Such a variation can be brought about by either a change in daily habits, such as shift working, or by moving to a different time zone. This has assumed greater significance in the jet age, due to the comparatively long time it takes to pick up a new Circadian rate.

Like a central-heating furnace with a timer the body's metabolic rate 'heats up' before the owner gets up, anticipating the need, and similarly at the end of the day it slows down some little time before turning in. The practical sign of this is that sweating (to take one example) is greater in the early morning than in the evening. Similarly more urine is secreted during the day than by night. An important application of this is that if a drug is being taken, insulin, for example, it is metabolised at different rates at different times of the 24-hour cycle.

Because the body clock is lazy, it finds it more difficult to catch up on time when travelling *against* the sun, i.e., West to East, than to lose time when travelling *with* the sun, East to West. Either way, this tends to upset established sleep patterns. More importantly, because it has no clock face to enable it to be 'read', the metabolic clock will be out of cycle with the destination time and habits, including timing on meals and type of food; also alcohol consumption, bowel habit, general alertness, together with diurnal temperature variations, pulse rate and blood pressure, as well as the efficacy of drugs and the condition of certain illnesses or disabilities whose containment depends on drugs. The symptoms of such illnesses can be exacerbated or even precipitated, for example, a diabetic coma induced, or, on a lesser scale, a fainting attack occurring, thus further disturbing the normal working of the body, and, more important for business purposes, unsettling mental processes, including concentration. All this can be summarised in one word: fatigue. It may not be recognised, for self-assessment will also be markedly impaired, in a manner not dissimilar to the effects of considerable quantities of alcohol.

The high-flyer of industry who boasts that he is not affected by jet aircraft travel is as much of a menace as the man who takes too much alcohol and proclaims that he can drive better. What happens in both instances is that judgement is impaired and, more importantly, self-judgement eliminated.

As in many other activities, the ability to overcome the effects of jet lag varies according to a number of factors. The three most important include age; older and younger people are more affected. However, so far as the young are concerned, the effect is more apparent than real as they tend to allow nature to take control. Indifferent or poor health adversely affects resistance to jet lag, as does exposure, in that repeated exposure would appear to confer at least a partial adaptation. Commercial aircrew adapt reasonably well, as do shift workers in workplaces. Temperaments are also thought to be relevant, and extroverts tend to adapt more quickly than introverts.

The tolerance to adaptation is also affected, not only by the direction of travel, as had been mentioned, but by the number of time zones covered. The body's clock would appear to be able to cope reasonably well with a rapid transition from one zone to another of 4–5 hours time zone change East to West, and 3–4 hours West to East. Anything in excess of these times will require about one day for each hour in excess of 5 hours time zone change, with up to 10 hours (5 days) to recover. After a flight in excess of 10 hours' time change, the body clock appears to 'flip' and meet itself coming the other way. When this happens, however, there is mental confusion as to what day it actually is!

Paradoxically, fatigue tends to nullify the effect of jet lag by overriding it. Fatigue is defined, physiologically, as 'a reduction in performance', and can result from excessive or extended activity, either of a mental or physical nature. In the context of this discussion, it is as though the body clock is running down and needs winding up again before it can resume its duties. The key to the rewinding lies in rest, sleep ideally, and the body clock will naturally pick up the local time when left to itself.

The explanation of this last statement can be found in an experiment carried out on oysters, in the days prior to jet travel. Already the speed of travel was beginning to outstrip the body's time clock's ability to keep up with the crossing of time zones. Oysters, like all molluscs, feed on a rising tide and their own 'hard case' clocks tend to be geared to a 25-hour day, to keep them synchronised with the local tides.

When some oysters were transported from England to North America, where not only the local time was different, but also the local tides were different, they were placed in tanks, not in the sea, and they clamped shut and remained shut for several days in some instances. As they gradually acclimatised to their new environment, they began to open and shut on a regular, but new cycle, which coincided with the local high tide, even though they were in tanks!

It should be noted that jet lag must be counted as a factor in stress, which should not be ignored completely if one is trying to live a little longer! (See stress factor in coronaries, Chapter Fourteen.)

Homo Sapiens as a Timekeeper

Whereas the body clock controls the timing of bodily functions and, as we have seen, tends to run on a natural 25-hour day (as does the moon, which historically tends to be linked with madness), man's ability to measure time has largely been replaced by chronometers, and so time measuring by the body is of little more than academic interest in the allegedly civilised world. Notwithstanding this, one can still gauge, albeit roughly, what time it is, but one is influenced by other bodily functions and needs, for example the need for food or sleep or some other biological function, and an estimate of 'time' is only accurate to about an hour or so.

When it comes to measuring elapsed time, man has poor ability, with an error marking of 30% or so. This is not surprising, as to estimate elapsed time one needs a unit by which to measure. Nature has not provided such a thing, and it has been left to man to invent one. Hence the second, the minute and the hour, for short-term elapsed time, and the day, week and month for longer periods. These can be conveniently marked by chronometers or calendars but there is no equivalent measure in physiological terms, only external clues like light and darkness, or temperature and similar indications, including seasonal changes, which measure positions in time but not elapsed time. The only exceptions are certain regular recurring happenings in the body, such as breathing or blinking, but even these are governed by other factors, breathing by chemicals in the bloodstream (oxygen, carbon dioxide), and blinking by a physical need to clean the eye at periodic intervals.

Whilst discussing inbuilt bodily mechanisms, we take our complex bodily functions far too much for granted, and are surprised when the body does not perform as well as we assume it will. In the complex human computer are many sophisticated devices. One is a 'direction finder' (not necessarily a compass, which works by reference to one of the Poles), and most living creatures have some form of location awareness, though the accuracy is variable from species to species, birds and fishes being the best from a navigational standpoint. Others are inaccurate from lack of use.

Human aviators tend to have a good 'bump of location'. There is anecdotal evidence to show that frequent travellers by any means, air or surface, seem to develop a sense of direction at a subconscious level, and can quickly orientate themselves when visiting a new location, subject to remaining on the same side of the Equator.

Why this should be is not clear, though it may well be similar to the migratory ability of birds in a way as yet to be explained. This navigational ability is fairly crude, and relates to the ability to tell north from south.

On crossing the Equator to an unaccustomed hemisphere this instinctive sense of direction becomes obscure by as much as 180 degrees; confusion ensues, towns turn round, the sun sets and rises in the wrong place. This does not appear to be related to wind direction (the wind goes round low pressure centres in a clockwise direction south of the equator), but attempts to navigate around a city and to learn the layout become difficult.

There is some suggestion that those afflicted with dyslexia and similar verbal disorientation problems are particularly affected, but more research is necessary before this can be confirmed. The better their ability to 'locate', the worse is the confusion in the opposite hemisphere.

Chapter Nine

It's Later Than You Think (or – Don't Forget to Wind up Your Clock)

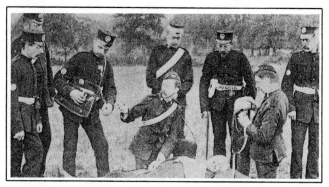

'Where there's hope – use a defibrillator.'
Anachronistic photograph of St John Ambulance at a training session.

Having, as it were, turned the tables on death by disposing of it at the beginning, rather than letting it have the final say as is more customary, we must not think we have disposed of the subject for ever, for death has a disquieting habit of turning up when least expected. For this reason, whilst not allowing this story to have a morbid preoccupation with the subject, we will keep a wary eye open and pay periodic homage by referring to it from time to time. Failure so to do may find us unprepared and bundled through that final trapdoor before we are ready, making an undignified exit in the process.

We will therefore note any milestones marking our progress through life, for noting them as they pass inevitably brings the 'final day' (judgement or otherwise) that much closer; this should not be in any way a morbid thought any more than the timing of any other event in our lives, from cooking to travelling on a journey.

The obvious way to estimate someone's age is by looking at them, although this is not always reliable. This is because after about the age of 40–45 an increasing number of people deviate from the 'index', looking older or younger either for natural reasons (weight increase, mannerisms, baldness) or because they have used artificial aids such as dyeing hair or using make-up.

Apart from appearances, the special senses of sight, hearing, and smell deteriorate at varying rates, and thus influence the age index as a hidden factor.

The age index can also be applied to a wide number of activities, such as various sports. The football index declines fairly steeply; golf less so, but this case is variable according to the degree of skill demanded.

Even sexual prowess has a place on the index, if a special one, but its impact is difficult to estimate without intimate knowledge, and even then a surprise may be in store!

Illness and disease will also distort and mislead, as, for example, Parkinson's disease, which can give a false impression of senility, whilst the underlying mental capabilities remain unaffected, a classic example of 'Does he take sugar?' syndrome. Similarly, the condition dysphasia (inability to speak) typically following a stroke, can cause great frustration and subsequent stress.

All Change?

A characteristic of ageing is an increasing reluctance to accept change of any sort. This reluctance applies to communities as much as to individuals. In both instances, progress, inhibited often in the name of preserving tradition or routine, can sometimes be dangerous, for example, trying to improve road layouts.

At a national level, dedication to the *status quo* became very apparent to me when I was on detachment duty with the United States Navy. In Britain, if some revolutionary proposal was made, involving a major change of policy on almost any matter, the response would be a tendency to ask, 'Why?', followed by many questions on the feasibility of the proposal. As a result, many good ideas have been abandoned unless supported by individuals.

FIGURE V: INDEX OF AGING

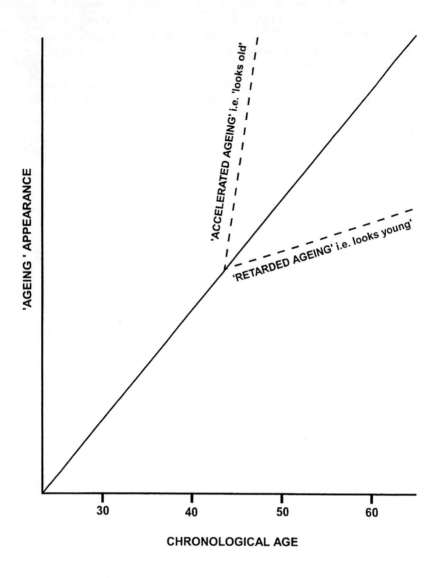

By contrast, if a similar proposal was made in America, the response tended to be, 'Why Not? Let's have a look and try it.' History is littered with ideas originating in Britain, but developed in America.

A reluctance to move into new circumstances may well be a factor in deciding whether to replace the royal yacht *Britannia*, and so maintain the *status quo* in principle as exemplified in the first line of the National Anthem.

Age and Change.

There is much to be said for the *status quo*, but not in absolute terms. 'Change' is anathema to the older person. Depending on the nature and impact of the proposed change, confusion and distress will vary from minimal to complete breakdown.

An elderly retired person leading a sedentary routine existence may resist change in a well-established routine, from a minor rearrangement of familiar furniture to the changing of a meal time or alteration of a visiting day.

The potential effects of such relatively minor changes should not be underestimated. In extreme cases they may uncover an already developing breakdown or dementia which has been kept at bay by the patient hanging on to familiar surroundings, faces, or a regular routine.

Some medical conditions can also make change more difficult for the sufferer to cope with. Pre-senile dementia (similar to Alzheimer's disease, but occurring at an earlier age), or a poor oxygen supply to the brain (bronchitis, heart problems, high blood pressure) can lead to confusion. All these may occur long before 'old age', but bring on a picture of 'old age' prematurely, inviting the comment: 'Hasn't so-and-so got old recently?' (See Figure V.)

An added danger is that illnesses are like medals: once you get one, a lot more seem to follow.

Some premature diseases can be self-induced by boredom with life. A relatively young person in regular employment of a routine nature which has not changed for many years may well show a falling-off in efficiency, even decadence, in his 50s. These very persons find it difficult to cope with the increasing need to change work conditions, calling for retraining in new skills and practices.

This leads to many finding themselves first unemployed, then unemployable in a rapidly changing work environment prejudiced against the 'older citizen' (which may now be misinterpreted as 'over 45'). The maximum time to spend in a single job might be considered to be 5 years.

The phrase 'it's later than you think' is applicable to the ageing process, but to the younger ambitious 'breadwinner' as well. Submitting to the temptation to switch jobs in search of a 'greener field' is to risk finding oneself playing the 'musical employment' game; when the rules allow the music to stop with embarrassing suddenness, the hitherto friendly world turns surprisingly unfriendly and can make you feel very old!

One day in Parliament Square, I was waiting for a friend whom I had not seen for years and was wondering how he might have changed, or indeed whether I would even recognise him. I looked up at Big Ben and it appeared to have stopped – or at least I couldn't see the hands actually moving. my friend was late, but my attention was diverted by a minor collision between two vehicles and the subsequent argument between the two drivers.

I looked at Big Ben again and noticed that the hands had moved on some ten minutes whilst I had watched the incident unfold. Reflecting on this incident, I spotted my friend, or, to be precise, I saw him getting off a bus, without seeing his face. I recognised him from the way he walked, as I had remembered him, and we greeted each other warmly, remarking on how well each looked, commenting 'you haven't changed at all'. Not true, of course, but then we are masters of self-deception. If we take the trouble to look at a large clock face closely – it doesn't have to be Big Ben – the small but discernible movement of the minute hand will be seen.

What then are the equivalent changes in ourselves, indiscernible from day to day, but nevertheless taking place? Are they additional lines or folds of the skin? Changes in underlying muscle mass or texture, causing the shape of the face to alter? Even colour, and hence make-up, can add to the deception, as can the colour of hair; even the way we move, be it speed, mode or even frequency of gestures, timbre of voice, speech modulation and so on.

I decided to run a simple experiment in the course of seeing patients (few of whom I visited a second time, owing to the nature of the medical examinations I was conducting), a considerable number of whom were totally blind; there were about 140 in total. Losing any particular sense, in this case, vision, causes the 'victim' (there can be compensations in becoming blind) to develop alternative ways of appraising his environment. Reckoning that these alternative ways would take some time to develop, I restricted my experiment to those who had been totally blind for at least five years, and matched them with equivalent persons with normal vision. I had some 60 persons in each of the two groups. Each subject was seen separately in the familiar surroundings of their own home, and it was explained that the purpose of the experiment was to ascertain how effectively people utilised their various senses to find out what was happening around them. In particular, I asked were they able to estimate somebody's age, and how did they do it?

At the time of the experiments I was in my 50s, had no grey hair, and was fairly fit and alert.

I alternated between a blind person (either sex) and someone with normal vision. I asked each subject to give a sincere estimate of my age. In both categories, a minority (about 10%) were so far out that their estimates were discarded (a higher proportion was in the group with normal vision, which I found surprising).

Of the remainder, those with normal vision *underestimated* my age by between four and seven years, some by up to 10 years.

In the case of the blind people, not only did they appear to give more thought to the matter but they were far more accurate, their estimates varying from two years younger to three years older than my true age.

As soon as this trend began emerging, I developed a list of supplementary questions as to how they arrived at their answers. The replies from those with vision were predictable, nearly all being along the lines of 'that is the age you look'.

The replies from the blind persons were much deeper and more subtle. The 'clues' which they used varied, but there was a common theme, mostly based on hearing, which assessed the pace of my walk, the character of my footsteps (one even referred to the degree of floor movement where I was walking, enabling them to estimate my weight), and a slight unsteadiness in my gait, due to my having damaged my semi-circular canals, and so affecting my balance! They also referred to the character of my handshake (tactile greetings are most important in any medical consultations, but especially so to blind persons), the timbre of my voice, my method of conducting the interrogation, and how much I was prepared to listen (a most important factor in clinical acumen, especially with older people).

In particular, though, more than one person identified my age by 'dating' idioms which I used, thus revealing that the very language we use is in itself going through an ageing process. One example cited was that I used the word 'wireless' instead of 'radio' on one occasion. Another picked up the word 'windscreen' (instead of 'windshield'). I felt that this was something of a 'reverse giveaway'!

Other examples of words noted by blind persons which helped them to 'date' ages included:

Running board (of a car).

Flagstones, now called paving stones.

A car dashboard, which is now called the fascia.

Motorists used to be 'summonsed'; now they 'get a ticket'.

Fountain pens are now ink pens, to distinguish them from biros.

'Carburettor' will soon be a dated term to young people.

To my surprise, a recent idiom used by youngsters under the age of about 22, is 'train station', as opposed to 'railway station', so that there is no confusion with 'bus station'. This may be indicative of a switch to long-distance bus travel.

Some buzz words have an even shorter cycle. 'Brilliant' became 'brill' around 1994, but reverted to 'brilliant' in 1995, making a small cohort of youngsters become precisely dated.

Older people still refer to 'telegrams', and very old people look forward to receiving their telegram from the Queen on their 100th birthday. Telegrams, as such, ceased in 1982.

There are many more examples, but the experiment led me to believe that blind people, and this could apply to other forms of physical handicap, utilised their other senses far more effectively, and were more 'observant' than their normally endowed colleagues, and thus were better informed.

Some changes might be temporary and reversible, such as dehydration, exhaustion, or even lack of sleep; others permanent, albeit susceptible to disguise.

Not all indications of ageing are physical; just as subtle are changes taking place to the personality that are of an intangible nature. Even more difficult to detect are mental changes, in part due to the inexorable dying-off of brain cells which takes place throughout life, without replacement. These changes (it would be incorrect to term them deteriorative or even degenerative, but rather morphogenetic) are even more difficult to identify than the physical changes caused by ageing. The subject can, and does, become subject to a variety of mental failings. This can be seen in Alzheimer's disease, where one symptom might take the form of an inability to tell the time from a watch. Should the sufferer be asked what time it is, he might well counter by saying, 'Why do you want to know?'

Wiliness in itself, though not restricted solely to old age, can be an index of ageing, or, as in the case of Alzheimer's disease, a manifestation of confusion. One case I recall was that of a physically fit woman in her mid-sixties who was found by her daughter going over the lawn with a vacuum cleaner. On consideration, this is a perfectly understandable action, given the similarities between a vacuum cleaner and a Flymo. Both machines require plugging into a source of electricity, the noises they make are not dissimilar, they are both pushed and pulled by hand, and remove unwanted material from a flat surface. Only the ability to identify the difference between the two tasks was lacking, with the result that the diagnosis became relatively simple, something which is not always so in an apparently rational conversation. Behaviour can remain superficially rational well into an advanced stage of such a disease.

Less discernible, and what might be termed physiological rather than pathological changes are taking place inside the brain, the central nervous system and special senses, but not at a uniform rate. These may be the consequence of a 'normal ageing' process. So deterioration is uneven and selective; some people retain an acute sense of hearing throughout their lives, whilst others become progressively hard of hearing; others, indeed a majority, grow grey, some at a very young age.

Whichever category you fall into, you cannot avoid the fact that ageing is inevitable from the moment of conception, and cannot be halted, much less reversed. So beware of getting too far 'off course', for the phrase 'mutton dressed as lamb' is no fable!

Are you getting older...? Or not really...? Maybe – just a bit? Do any of the following statements seem just a little familiar? If so, can you explain why... or does the cap fit? The actual progress of ageing is well marked with tell-tale signs:

1) How young the policemen seem (or bus drivers, grandmothers, or for that matter almost anyone!). The next stage of this phenomena (usually when one has reached 70+) is that when regarding policemen, or officers in one's old regiment, they don't look unduly young! The explanation for this is that in one's own estimation, after about 65 one ceases to get older, or so it seems, and one even thinks of 'self' getting younger! It's probably important for older people to celebrate their birthdays, as a salutary reminder that they are getting older.

2) A tendency to look first at the 'death columns' in the papers, before marriages and births. Then the latter are skipped altogether. After the age of 75, a further change occurs, with declining interest in the deaths column. This is because the peak of deaths takes place at the age of 75, so that an increasing number of one's contemporaries have died, and so fewer left to watch for.

3) How much faster other cars seem to be going nowadays ('Why is everyone so impatient? No consideration or manners!').

4) 'What is the world coming to?'

5) 'I seem to be the first into a public lavatory, but always take longer than anybody else, and am probably the last to leave.'

6) 'Tom [or Dick or Harry] seems to be getting very frail nowadays.'

7) 'The drinks one gets in pubs seem so much weaker nowadays.'

8) 'These modern clothes – they seem to lose their shape so.'

9) In my own case: when I reached 50 I could no longer 'greet' the face I saw in the mirror each morning and so took to shaving in the bath. However, this, ostrich-like, only served to put off the day, so that the shock was greater when I did see my face in photographs.

10) On qualifying for my senior citizen reduced-fare rail card (at 60), the ticket inspectors would always ask for confirmation of my age; they no longer do!

11) They use smaller print nowadays.

12) My elderly patients were in the habit of referring to me as 'that nice young man': no more!

13) That pleasant old-world habit of addressing one as 'sir' seems to be on the increase!

14) 'Don't confuse me with the facts.'

To the speaker, the above statement is simply a way of stating his position, but more probably is pathogenetic of either:

a) Advancing years and/or:

b) That, having developed his 'task' (either his own business, or over many years a department in an organisation), the demands of the now sophisticated 'task' have outgrown his executive capability. Metaphorically, he is now 'hanging on for dear life' and no longer in control of either the 'task' or his own destiny. This is not only potentially damaging for both the individual and the organisation, but a situation which calls for considerable tact in knowing how to rectify the position. This is similar to older people becoming absent-minded, but is potentially more dangerous, as executive command and responsibility may be involved.

The final shock for me came one day when, travelling on a No. 11 bus in London, a Chelsea pensioner, in his red hospital uniform, offered me his seat. Mortified, I declined, muttering something about getting off at the next stop (I wasn't). Then he said, "Well, so am I." Committed, we both got off; he went into the Chelsea Hospital, and I had to wait for the next bus! I wasn't completely mollified when I learned later that one qualifies to be an in-pensioner at the age of 60.

There is, however, a twist in the tale. When I started to recount this story some years ago it could always be relied upon to raise a laugh. However, just recently, in my mid 70s, I had to address an audience of several hundred people and decided to lighten the day a little by recounting my old story. As I began, I realised that my audience were relatively young, many in their mid 40s or 50s. As I finished, there was an embarrassed silence with scarcely a murmur.

I then realised the awful truth: they could not see anything unusual in somebody, anybody, offering a seat to an old man! I had taken a sudden quantum leap into old age!

Of course, after a few days, I had convinced myself that the logical explanation for the 'being offered a seat' story was that the modern sense of humour had shifted and that such a story was no longer appropriate for, nor appreciated by youngsters. However, my smugness was given a further blow, when, just recently, a letter was forwarded from my publisher of *Hippocrates RN*. It started harmlessly enough expressing appreciation, and saying how much the writer had enjoyed it. Of course, my vanity was touched and I warmed to the unknown letter writer, but then I came upon a postscript in the letter which read: '...please pass this letter on to Dr Ellis – if he is still with us...'!

These uncomfortable home truths come sometimes from unexpected quarters: I am fortunate to have a wonderful doctor as my GP, Clarissa Fabre. She is, of course, far too young to be the senior partner, but there it is, and she is. I had occasion to be referred by Clarissa to a consultant for some minor 'tidying up'. Some time later, sitting in Clarissa's surgery on another matter, I noticed an impish look in her eye when she suggested I might be interested in seeing my notes, turning them towards me. The top document was a letter from the consultant which began.

> *Dear Dr Fabre,*
>
> *Thank you for sending me this charming, eccentric, elderly gentleman...*

'Be Prepared'

That old Baden-Powell motto, though no longer followed, has a place in modern living: an enthusiastic (for what I'm not revealing) friend of mine used to say, "I always wear a clean pair of underpants every day, I never know when I might find myself in a situation when somebody might take them off." (He died unexpectedly from a massive coronary thrombosis shortly afterwards – he was found sitting on the loo!). Ironically, a sudden 'call to stool' is a common forewarning of an imminent sudden heart attack (or pulmonary embolus), but that is no justification for deferring a call to nature; it will get you in the end.

'It's All in the Mind'

If you can dream – and not make dreams your master;
If you can think – and not make your thoughts your aim.

Rudyard Kipling

It's time for a man to take the long, long sleep, when his
mind makes appointments which the body can't keep.

Anon

Spare a thought for the tramp in the following story. He had
reached an age when any pleasure that he might partake in was
wholly in his mind, rather than in reality. Even this 'perchance to
dream' philosophy is not without its attendant dangers though!

Alas, this old man had partaken of a couple of 'jars' too many, so
that, one fine balmy evening, by the time he went to seek out his
customary bench on the Embankment, they had all been occupied.
Exhausted, he had little energy left to search further afield, so
climbed up on to the four-foot wide embankment, covered himself as
best he could with his newspapers, and was soon moving into that
twilight sleep phase, lulled by the gentle sounds of the Thames far
below him.

He became aware that somebody was approaching him, and,
fearing the police, he opened one eye, to observe somebody dressed
in a chauffeur's uniform, with a Rolls Royce parked beside the kerb
behind him.

"Excuse me, my man, but m'lady saw you settling down, and
wonders if you might not be more comfortable in her spare room in
Dolphin Square – it's just round the corner."

Hardly believing his good fortune, the tramp, abandoning his
newspaper blankets to the river, scrambled down and, following the
chauffeur, climbed into the back of the Rolls alongside a well-
endowed redhead, who welcomed him with a smile and suggested he
would certainly have a better night where they were going.

Arriving at Dolphin Square, they got out of the car, and were
admitted to the penthouse suite by a footman.

"Albert, show my guest to the pink room." And with a brisk
"Have a pleasant night," she was gone.

The tramp was shown into the pink room, adequately and
appropriately furnished with a large double bed with a pair of pink
silk pyjamas laid out.

114

Undressing, the tramp gladly climbed into bed, and – for the second time within an hour, was just dropping off to sleep, when the door opened, and he saw with great anticipation, 'm'lady' coming in, dressed in an exotic and provocatively worn full-length nightdress.

As she made to get into bed, she whispered, "Move over, I'm joining you."

The tramp obligingly moved over, and... fell thirty feet into the Thames.

What a pity, but... such is life... full of surprises... and he'd thrown his newspapers away!

The Wrong Career – as a Stress Factor.

Career planning starts early: as good foundations are essential in building, so early training of the mind ('learning how to learn') is critical to enable formal learning to follow smoothly when embarking upon the acquisition of formal qualifications for a career.

Career qualifications may be either constrictive or open. The former make for easy access to other careers or for switching in mid-career from one discipline to another with minimal difficulty.

Examples of constrictive qualifications include: medicine and dentistry (restricting switching only from one speciality to another, and even this can pose problems unless done early), commercial flying, very constricting even from airborne duties to ground duties, with executive appointments virtually unheard of. Other careers difficult to leave include: the armed forces (especially if left till late), architecture, and, surprisingly, a career in banking.

Open qualifications include legal (especially suited to political careers, where an ability to make quick assessments and to speak publicly is invaluable). In today's litigious society, when legal opinions are frequently resorted to, to be legally correct is often given a higher priority than pragmatism, though in the end the two may well be found, at a price, to be mutually compatible.

Perhaps the best of all open qualifications are those that have no qualifying attributes at all, but merely indicate a good, well-trained brain, achievements something like a First in Classics, or Greats, or some similar obscure subject!

This, coupled with that sometimes infuriating trait of not saying very much, will ensure a smooth, steady progression with the steady collection of a number of non-executive directorships, each one carrying with it a mythical reputation until appropriate honours become inevitable, making the original qualifications of little more than academic interest.

Once the mind is trained to think, it is more likely to remain supple and adaptable to an older age and so slow down the ageing processes. A spring in the footstep and sparkle of the mind will be reflected in the eyes, if only to avoid stepping in the excreta left by the dogs on the pavement, or in the human equivalent as you progress through life's jungle!

Given a basic education as so described, the day of the jack of all trades is returning, with one who recognises the brief openings of 'opportunity doors' as they occur in life, discerning those that merely have a brightly illuminated porch but nothing of substance beyond. It is tempting to leave the wide open road for the relative security of a near zoological garden safety environment. Professionals such as pathologists, psychiatrists, those in the higher echelon of the judiciary, some accountancy sinecures and some remote government departments come into this category, but carry the musty aroma of stultification which has a high associated risk of pomposity and accelerated ageing. This can be examined along selected reaches of golf clubs, some voluntary callings, any obscure habitat calling for committees, or occasional gatherings, especially if such gatherings call for the donning of uniforms (or similar) and the diffident wearing of medals or other adornments, calculated to reinforce a sometimes faded habit of acknowledging reverence. Military titles even if obsolete, are especially encouraged. Indeed, obsolescence is especially welcomed, as it encourages speculation as to the title's precise meaning: 'Surgeon General' is one such title, as is 'Barber Surgeon', though even a subsequent extended discussion leaves one little the wiser.

Barristers especially, until they get elevated, keep in practice at being 'smart', especially in their often clever use of precise English, at the expense of their supposed seniors and betters.

Some human characteristics do become more refined with advancing years; one such is the ability to be romantic.

When I visited elderly lady patients (see Chapter Twelve) I was always impressed with the reaction when I took their hands to feel their pulses. Looking into their eyes, one could see a young girl there. Older ladies are committed romantics, and it was touching to see how they returned to memories of their youth.

I once mentioned this to a nursing sister, and she said that she had noticed the same thing about elderly men, so maybe it is a manifestation of age. It reinforced my belief that there are many little pleasures to be had from the evening of life.

'I Don't Think That's Quite What I Meant'

Beauty is the eye of the beholder

Molly Bawn, 1878

When I met Jean, now my wife, I was nearly 70, and, you may say, I was old enough to have known better – I became aware that I was still capable of sensing a romantic touch. I should also have remembered the wisdom of thinking something through before speaking. Unfortunately, on this occasion I didn't.

We had not known one another for very long, but I had already suspected that we were likely to spend our future together. Jean was already steeling herself psychologically for her 70th birthday, and we were visiting some friends near Durban, in South Africa.

One evening, we were dining in a restaurant overlooking the Indian Ocean, on which the full moon's reflection was shimmering. It was a romantic evening, and called for an appropriate word, as I gazed into Jean's face, gently lit up by the single candle, which was flickering in the slight breeze. I suppose I ought to say that the orchestra was playing quietly in the background, but that would be a tale too far! Nevertheless, I took her hand (*that* was all right – quite appropriate). Then I heard myself speak, as though it was somebody else, and, with horror, heard this 'disembodied voice' pronounce, "You couldn't look any older than you do tonight," and then, in an effort to put it right, again I heard, "I think I meant to say – you couldn't look any younger!"

Perhaps it was about then that I realised what a lovely personality Jean is, as she replied, "I know what you are *trying* to say – let's just enjoy the view."

There was a second occasion, when I was discussing the Index of Ageing at a dinner party, and was defending a view about how lucky some people could be if they didn't look any more than the Index. Attempting to make my point with the heavily made-up lady on my right, I said at a point when there was one of those silences, "Well, you certainly look *your* age."

I seem to recollect that it was one of those occasions when we didn't stay too late.

'Ageing' – A Constructive Thought:

So far, the process of ageing has been discussed as though it was a single entity, a process along the pathway of life without reference to other factors, including changes on that pathway. These very changes, especially if significant and rapid, are as important in 'dating' persons as their own ageing process.

The ability to perform in society depends not only on how old you are, but also how conversant you are with today's practices. There are two factors to consider: your age, and fitness for your age.

On the second of these, if you have just re-joined society (work or socially) because, for example, you have been ill, unemployed for whatever reason for some years, have been abroad, have immigrated into a country, or if you have emigrated to a new country with a different culture, or even simply a foreign language, you may not be conversant with the usual moves.

Irrespective of your age, any of these factors are going to put you at some disadvantage. The older you are when undergoing these changes the more difficult it will be to adapt to the new conditions for two reasons:

1) Adaptability becomes more difficult with age.

2) This difficulty is increased if an old skill or habit has to be unlearned or modified, hence my own 'experiment' in re-learning to fly.

A Square End – the Optimum Finish to Life

Progressive deterioration of both physical and certain mental faculties commences alarmingly early in life, and it is only experience that maintains the quality of life at an acceptable level. Notwithstanding this, life's quality tends to fall off unacceptably early for too many persons. This, compounded with an inability to make a contribution to society may explain the persistent rise in crime today, when many find themselves unable and unqualified to make any contribution to society.

FIGURE VI: QUALITY OF LIFE

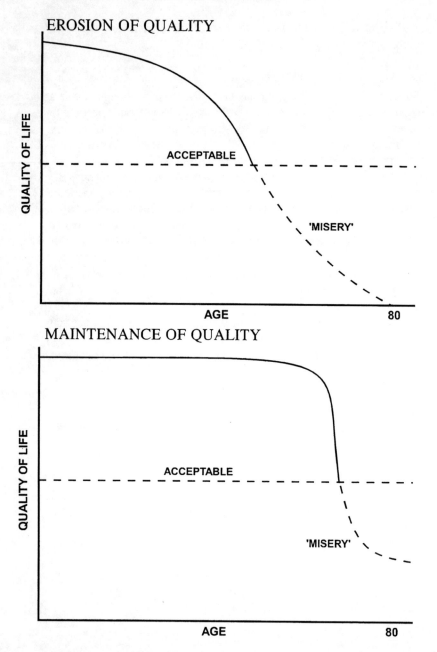

EROSION OF QUALITY

QUALITY OF LIFE

ACCEPTABLE

'MISERY'

AGE   80

MAINTENANCE OF QUALITY

QUALITY OF LIFE

ACCEPTABLE

'MISERY'

AGE   80

Put in graphic form, (see Figure VI), the fall-off in life's qualities may well result in a feeling of hopelessness at an early age, aggravated by a feeling of abandonment by society, high unemployment, insecurity even whilst in employment, and eventually insecurity amongst one's fellow beings – the whole being fanned by a monetary shortage.

The economic implications of this scenario are discussed elsewhere, but will stand repetition as the Government is beginning to address the growing imbalance between the contributing workers and the expanding 'leisured' class, whose numbers are swollen by early retirement and redundancies.

Re-employment of the retired population at cost-effective rates and re-categorising the retired and re-employed persons into a new 'remploy' category would be both tax- and cost-effective if the 'remployed' were given particular privileges as regards working hours and wage rates. These measures, together with the general health guidelines suggested in this book, would make a major contribution towards achieving a 'square end' to life.

Chapter Ten

Do You Want to Live a Little Longer?

It could be that, after reading this book, you may have revised your ambitions, but do you want to continue for... a *little* longer? A *lot* longer? Or are you ready to fade away during the next few days?

This is not an easy question to answer. It will vary according to your age, your state of health, your personal circumstances, your contentment or unhappiness and a host of other factors which together make up that difficult thing to define or even to measure: 'quality of life'.

Perhaps it might be helpful, therefore, if the various factors are analysed.

Your Design Life

This varies from creature to creature; a mayfly is designed to live for a single day, whereas a crocodile is believed to be capable of living for well over 100 years.

Remember that, although you are most unlikely to reach it, your design life is approximately 125 years, so at the point of death *much* of your body will be still relatively serviceable!

Expectation of Life.

This statistic is widely misused. For example, it is often stated that man's expectation of life has doubled in the last 100 years. This is statistically true, but misleading. The statistic refers to the life expectancy of a newly born babe, whose ambitions for his or her future are strictly limited to such things as the next meal or the state of his or her nappy, and similar mundane things.

At the beginning of the century he should have been much more concerned as to whether he was going to survive the next few weeks or not, for the risk of neonatal death was very real, and it was this factor which restricted the life expectancy. Once the infant had survived the first ten years or so, his life expectancy dramatically increased and was not far short of that of a similarly aged child today. This is entirely due to neonatal deaths having been virtually eliminated. It is often said that 'people live longer nowadays', which is just as misleading. It is simply that there are more older people around because there was a 'bulge' (cohort) in the numbers being born in the first part of this century, and those same people have now become older. For a variety of reasons, the birth rate has dropped off in the second half of this century, bringing in its wake the problem of how the surfeit of 'old' people are to be provided for by the diminishing numbers of 'young'uns'.

As we can see, during the ninth decade of life, the 'carrot' element of the 'carrot and stick' comes into play, epitomising Jonathan Swift's picture of how death can become – apparently – elusive! Interestingly, members of the clergy are amongst the longest living – paradoxically, the arrival at the 'promised land' is seriously delayed!

FIGURE VII: THE LONG LIFE TABLE
Figures refer to European males – females add approximately 4 years.

PRESENT AGE	LIFE EXPECTANCY	PRESENT AGE	LIFE EXPECTANCY
15	75.57	27	76.38
16	75.61	28	76.44
17	75.67	29	76.50
18	75.73	30	76.56
19	75.80	31	76.61
20	75.88	32	76.66
21	75.95	33	76.71
22	76.03	34	76.76
23	76.10	35	76.80
24	76.18	36	76.85
25	76.25	37	76.90
26	76.32	38	76.95

PRESENT AGE	LIFE EXPECTANCY	PRESENT AGE	LIFE EXPECTANCY
39	77.00	51	78.00
40	77.06	52	78.13
41	77.12	53	78.27
42	77.18	54	78.42
43	77.24	55	78.58
44	77.31	56	78.75
45	77.39	57	78.93
46	77.47	58	79.12
47	77.56	59	79.32
48	77.66	60	79.54
49	77.76	61	79.77
50	77.88	62	80.01

PRESENT AGE	LIFE EXPECTANCY	PRESENT AGE	LIFE EXPECTANCY
63	80.27	75	84.66
64	80.54	76	85.15
65	80.83	77	85.65
66	81.14	78	86.17
67	81.46	79	86.71
68	81.80	80	87.27
69	82.15	81	87.85
70	82.53	82	88.65
71	82.92	83	89.07
72	83.33	84	89.70
73	83.76	85	90.35
74	84.20	86	91.02

PRESENT AGE	LIFE EXPECTANCY	PRESENT AGE	LIFE EXPECTANCY
87	91.71	94	96.96
88	92.42	95	97.74
89	93.14	96	98.51
90	93.88	97	99.26
91	94.64	98	99.97
92	95.50	99	100.62
93	96.18	100	101.16

Source: *Medical Selection of Life Risks* by R.D.C Brackenridge and W. John Elder.

Politicians and certain others who should know better, seem to find it convenient to place anyone over the age of 70 into a special category labelled 'unrepairable and to be given palliative medical treatment only – supplemented by liberal doses of sedation if necessary'. Future voting powers of such categories should, however, be noted. Consider the following 'cocktail' of UK statistics:

A.   1951:   There were 300 persons over 100.
      2011:   There will be in excess of 25,000 people over 100
                (an increase of over 1000%).
      1961:   There were 300,000 persons over 85.
      2012:   There will be 1.5 million people over 85.

But today, over 700,000 people suffer from some form of dementia – mostly in the older age groups.

B.   Increasing Life Expectancy

Year	Male	Female
1941	59.0	64.0
1951	65.6	70.4
1961	67.9	73.6
1971	69.1	75.3
1981	70.9	76.9
1991	73.2	78.7

Conclusion

Increasing life expectancy plays only a small part in the growth in the numbers of the elderly – it is simply that there is a cohort of 'elderly' people. But... the effect on the economy could be devastating:

C.   1961:   There were 8 million pensioners.
      2031:   There will be 16 million pensioners.

By 2000, those over 50 will control over 80% of the country's wealth.

Political expediency has put this problem to one side, but not for long. Shifting the 'indexing' of pensioners from 'earnings related' to 'cost of living' slowed the burden, but only temporarily, for retiring people will face an ever-increasing fall in their living standards upon retirement. It would be a political mistake of the first magnitude to ignore this potential of ability and wisdom, for a considerable number of persons over the age of 65 are physically able, mentally alert, and independent, able to make a contribution to society as opportunities open.

It is disheartening for those people who do not feel or consider themselves to be 'old' to be bombarded with newspaper articles referring to 'caring for the elderly' and the like. It would be more constructive to be encouraged on how much the elderly might contribute, having cared for themselves, for being reminded of 'being old' is a sure recipe for curtailing life itself.

In my collection of case histories of over 10,000 persons – mostly from the upper age groups (7.8% over 90), one in particular comes to mind – an ex-pilot aged 73, who regained his pilot's licence after an absence from flying lasting over 30 years. His only disappointment was that it took him over 5 hours to go 'solo' – compared with just over 4 hours when he first started in 1946!

As a gerontologist (a student of the ageing process) I do not wish to be confused with a geriatrician who cares for old people. I would not like my own role to become muddled with the wrong group, or even mistaken for one of them!

For practical purposes, I would suggest the following definitions:

Middle age: 45 – 65
'Elderly':   65 – 85
'Old':   over 85
'Seriously old':   over 90

The term 'geriatric' should be reserved to describe a medical condition – not a person's age. As a maxim, I would quote that eminent physician, Denis Burkitt:

> *Attitudes are more important than abilities.*
> *Motives are more important than methods.*
> *Character is more important than cleverness.*
> *Perseverance is more important than power.*
> *And the heart takes precedence over the head.*

Ageing: Skill and Employability

The growing imbalance between the providers in a nation (see above) – i.e., the employed population, and the consumers (the retired and the unemployed) will soon reach crisis point – within the next ten years. It is largely responsible for the growing, and soon to be unsustainable levels prevailing, and, in itself, a very threat to the stability of society. Encouraging the retired (which now includes the 'early retired') to take up employment within the scope of their capabilities once more (conditional on their locality; part-, or full-time; incentives offered etc.) would make a substantial contribution towards closing the 'pension gap'.

Remuneration could be related to a pension datum point (65), and would be largely self-funding.

Examples: Manual labourers could be switched to caretaking.

Ex-policemen could undertake clerical duties, leaving the younger officers to concentrate on the more energetic, and dangerous tasks.

It would, however, be at the higher 'executive' or board levels where most benefit might accrue. However, the threat of an older director to a chief executive would have to be guarded against, so the advocate, to give an interim title, would have no responsibility except consultancy, nor any power – the chief executive would elect to listen or not – as he chose – to views stemming from 'wisdom'. One very essential ingredient, the 'calculated risk' decision, would thus be left in play – but this very quality – so essential in arriving at business policy decisions – begins to ebb away in the middle 50s, and must be left unfettered.

This area requires considerable thought to realise its potential. A start might be made by persuading the charity Help the Aged to modify its title to: LET THE AGED HELP.

The Quality of Life.

This embraces a number of widely diverse matters:

a) Health: This must rank high on the list, or to be accurate, the lack of it must; this will depend on whether any affliction is static, and can therefore be tolerated or one's lifestyle adapted. If the affliction is progressive, and therefore possibly terminal and finite, some might elect not to live out the maximum remaining months (or even years).

b) Happiness (or paucity thereof): This also depends on a number of factors, and might include grief, perhaps following the loss of a loved one or companion on whom one has become dependent, or even the loss of a household pet. The ability to overcome the effects of grief will decline with age, for the older we are, the less resilient we become. Thus, a long relationship with another person can become too ingrained, making it difficult or impossible to adopt a suddenly imposed independent lifestyle, the result being a life-threatening situation.

c) Material Sufficiency: The suggestion that 'money cannot buy happiness' wears a bit thin in today's materialistic world, and a sufficiency of cash must be listed as essential; this is borne out by the varying life expectancy between the different socio-economic groups. Please refer to Chapter Seven before wishing or striving to acquire a glut of riches. There is often a heavy price to be paid for such acquisitions.

d) Age: In the younger person the fundamental instinct to continue to survive runs most strongly. Note that it is 'survival', rather than a will to live; thus, adrenaline is the life-saver rather than the way of life. In these early years there is a paradox, for, although the will to survive is strong, there is also a strong inclination to take risks and to become exposed to life-threatening events, which may take the form of anything from parachuting to white water rafting. In the absence of such opportunities, youngsters manufacture scenarios accounting for considerable excursions into crime of one form or another. This might well be termed the 'peace penalty', for which service in one of the armed forces provided a natural safety valve.

It is no coincidence that the suicide rate, especially amongst younger people, has risen dramatically in recent years. The reasons are not clear, but manifestly the quality of life for this sad group of people had become unacceptable. It might be either of two extremes: that life had become too stressful and demanding, to the extent that the victim felt unable to cope or measure up to this demand, or conversely, that life did not offer a sufficient challenge, thus resulting in frustration. Both extremes could explain the alternative option of turning to crime. It is tempting to believe that a solution could lie in some form of national service for 12–18 months, which would offer an outlet for enterprise within the capability of the 'patient', for that is what these unfortunate people are.

If the old form of military national service is no longer practical, the net cost of some form of 'service to the nation', after deducting the outlay of the various forms of social security 'benefits' (including the administration costs thereof), must be affordable. One suggestion is that it might take the form of a period of service in the county police force or in the fire service, for at least that would introduce discipline and succour the more adventurously inclined.

How Much Longer and How Much Will You Strive to Live?

The will to live (as well as the desire) both diminish progressively with advancing years; apart from illness, there is no sudden evaporation of this will but just a weakening in resolve.

Having eliminated the neo-natal bulge (see Figure VIII – area A), the next target in the battle to survive is the 'middle-aged spread', affecting the 45–65s (area B).

Nineteen out of every hundred (presumably healthy) males aged 45 will die before reaching 65. Are *YOU* ready?

As the will to live still beats strongly amongst those at risk in the 45–65 age bracket, what steps might one take to avoid those life-threatening illnesses? In practice quite a lot, for they are the largest group of 'voluntary' illnesses during the whole lifespan, and are caused by smoking (responsible for 25%-33% of all deaths, mostly in the prime of life), road traffic accidents, coronaries and suicides.

These are examples where positive preventive measures to avoid premature death would pay off.

I also wondered if there might be any negative measures: how about flying? Highly dangerous, and to be avoided some might think, but of course we all know that flying is as safe as... Well is it?

To find out, I looked for statistics relating to flying safety, and, not unexpectedly, it depended how, and with what airline, and where you choose to fly. This was revealed in *Fortune* magazine.

I found that during 1992, 54 people died in air crashes in the United States, a rate of 0.6 deaths per million departures from an airport. Indeed, it was positively a guarantee for avoiding death when this figure of 54 deaths due to flying was compared to figures showing that no fewer than 318 Americans died whilst taking a bath, 6,500 died whilst crossing the road, and some 7,000 unfortunate souls were murdered by their spouses.

FIGURE VIII: SECOND BATTLE OF THE BULGE

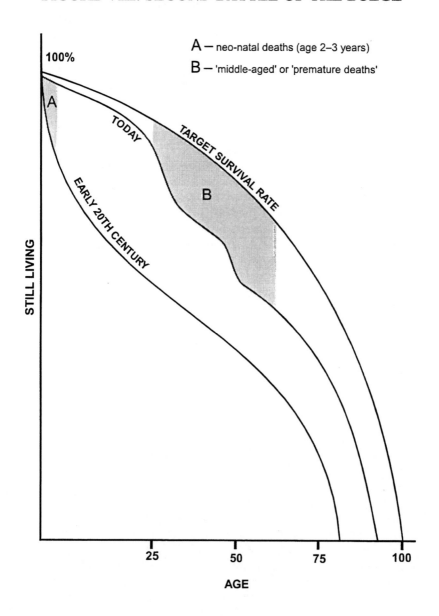

A — neo-natal deaths (age 2–3 years)
B — 'middle-aged' or 'premature deaths'

100%

TODAY

TARGET SURVIVAL RATE

EARLY 20TH CENTURY

STILL LIVING

AGE

25   50   75   100

Similar statistics for the Western world are published. Supposing you have a sudden yen to see the Taj Mahal: you had better think twice before rushing out to buy that air ticket from the local bucket shop, and it is important to choose your carrier with care. You may be well impressed by Indian Airlines, which, with a death rate of 1.58 per million departures compares favourably with the overall rate for Asia as a whole (2.97). You might indeed have an interesting flight, as happened to an Indian Airbus A320 in 1990, whose crew, on a day with good visibility, missed the arrival runway by 2,000 feet, and landed on a golf course (interesting if you're a golfer; less so for the others!). They managed to get airborne again, but on the next approach landed before even reaching the runway, and ended by ploughing into a brick wall, killing 92 people.

A flight does not have to finish in a mass of tangled metal and fatalities to be eventful; many events take place without the passengers even being aware that anything untoward has happened, or nearly has, or even might have done.

I well recall flying on a local flight into Tierra de Fuego, at the southernmost tip of South America. I was taking a keen interest, mindful that the death rate from flying accidents for South America is amongst the highest in the world (4.87 per million departures). We were flying in a small twin-engined aircraft, unpressurised, confirmed, as I could see the sea far below through a gap in the floorboards! We seemed to continue climbing for an unusually long time.

For this I was thankful as there are some lethally high mountains in this part of the world. This relief was offset by my observing that the two pilots, whom I could see through the open door leading to the flight deck, seemed to spend more time peering anxiously outside as we flew in and out of cloud. This was presumably to see where the mountain peaks were, rather than flying on their instruments which would have been more reliable then visual checkings in cloud!

I was also concerned as we had a number of older passengers, including one with a heart ailment; I glanced at her, and noticed that her lips were turning a delightful shade of blue, and not due to make-up, or cold. Our guide was Sybil Sassoon, an old friend of mine, and I knew that she always carried a portable barograph with her. I asked her what the pressure was, and with a simple calculation, I deduced we were by now flying at some 14,000 feet, and still climbing. I expressed my concern to Sybil for the welfare of the passengers, and was not reassured when I noticed that the pilot was wearing an oxygen mask (in another way I was relieved). At the time I thought I could recall a flying story with a not dissimilar theme, something about there not being enough parachutes to go round, but the shortage of oxygen was already beginning to cloud my memory.

Sybil thought for a minute and looked around at her charges.

"Oh, they seem quite happy; most of them are asleep."

"Asleep, be damned," I replied. "They're not asleep, they're unconscious!" At that moment, thank goodness, we commenced descending, and I was most relieved when we landed at our destination and everyone woke up!

One might postulate that such happenings put the Prince of Wales' 'arrival' on a Scottish island runway into perspective, and restores a modicum of confidence in his skill as a pilot. After all, it used to be said in the Royal Air Force that a landing is acceptable if everyone can walk away from it. However skilled one is, we all make mistakes at some time, though usually without the attendant publicity.

Occasionally, a scheduled flight can sow seeds of doubt before the flight has even thought of commencing; one such moment of doubt comes to mind, which occurred in Nigeria.

I was flying from Lagos to Cotonou, in the neighbouring country of Benin, and although it was only some sixty miles away, the flight had the status of an international departure. As I waited for the flight to be called, I reflected nervously that one was twenty times as likely to be killed flying in these parts as in North America. Armed with this daunting statistic, I was hardly reassured when I heard the flight called with directions 'to proceed to a waiting Land-Rover and be taken to a remote corner of the airfield where the aircraft was parked and would depart in due course'.

Proceeding around the perimeter track (I was, apparently, the only passenger), I noticed a passenger jet aircraft parked by itself. Some maintenance men were pulling hunks of palm leaves and branches out of the flaps, which were fully extended. I enquired what they were doing, suggesting perhaps that it was only used for fire-fighting and that the jungle was beginning to repossess it. My jolly black driver denied this and explained that the aircraft had arrived earlier on a scheduled service, but had 'got a little low' during the approach for landing. My apprehension was interrupted by our arriving at the aircraft – an ancient DC3 (Dakota).

As we drew up at the apparently deserted aircraft, my black driver wished me a 'fortunate flight'! – adding that any other passengers who could be found would be rounded up.

The sun was hot so I ventured up the wobbly aluminium ladder into the back of the aircraft. It had one occupant, an Arab Sheikh, dressed in long, flowing white robes. He did not speak, and I settled down in one of the seats. The Dakota was the workhorse of World War II with a good record for safety, and, having flown one, I was familiar with its eccentricities. One of these was that, when sitting on the ground, the nose was high up in the air, and it was quite a climb to go from the rear entrance door up to the pilot's flight deck.

After some time, I became aware that somebody else was climbing aboard, and I turned round to see a white man with a long flowing white beard ('Father Time' crossed my mind), in an official-looking uniform, start laboriously walking up the aisle of the plane. He was dressed in white shorts, white stockings, and cap, clearly the badge of the airline, and was probably attaching himself to this flight. The effort to get to the cockpit had made him rather short of breath.

Feeling thirsty, I said kindly, "Gracious, you look far too old to be a steward, but could I have some water please?"

He paused as if to regain his breath, before snapping, "I am too old to be clambering up and down this piece of antiquity, serving drinks, however, I'm not the steward, in fact we don't have one; I'm the pilot."

With that, he disappeared into the front, and, before I had recovered or had time to change my mind, he had started the engines, and we were off at considerable speed. I formed the impression that he could well have been the original DC3 test pilot!

I tightened my safety-belt another notch. Was it my imagination that it was constructed of elastic material or was I just getting nervous?

Significant numbers of passengers still feel varying degrees of apprehension over the prospect of a forthcoming flight. Symptoms range from mild nervousness to frank terror. Cynical as it may appear, possibly motivated by commercial self-interest, several airlines offer an introductory familiarisation course to flying, with talks, consultations, and finishing with a brief flight. Results of this policy are not published. Possibly from deference to those of an imaginative disposition, self-service machines offering life cover insurance are no longer prominently placed for the convenience of prospective passengers at the departure gates! On the other hand, discreet notices offering facilities for praying are still scattered around the departure areas.

Further reflecting on the widespread incidence of advertising of every type and for every product – including travel sickness remedies – one trade is conspicuous by its absence at airports: funeral directors.

Considering, in more general terms, the decor of airports, and with memories of my medical practice days, it does seem singularly inappropriate for departure gates to be associated with the word 'terminal', an unfortunate connotation for the more imaginative, and potentially nervous passenger.

The ocean-going equivalent buildings are much more tactfully described as 'docks' or 'quays' – at least you would only have to swim, should the worst come to the worst.

Once installed in your aircraft seat, you probably feel the worst is over, and, if fortunate, have a drink in your hand, if not in your stomach. You settle back, listen to the engines winding up, and, after 'push-out' – what could that imply? – you are reassured by a few words of encouragement from a disembodied voice, as you rattle towards what you hope is the downwind end of the runway. (Goodness, will there be sufficient fuel to get all the way?)

At the outset of one flight I had in the American mid-west, we seemed to wait for an interminably long while at the 'holding' point, prior to obtaining take-off clearance, when the pilot, in an inimitable Southern drawl, announced that he was sorry for the delay, but that 'we shall be taking off momentarily': I called for another gin and tonic! Have a good flight.

During the middle phase in life, apart from steps taken to avoid premature death, people do not generally think about the 'ultimate' death age; when asked, they tend to reply without much thought and mention mid to late 70s as being a 'good innings'.

Several important things have emerged from my own researches on the matter:

First, that retirement is a major milestone in life and arguably can be the most difficult 'career' of one's life. If one can avoid the 'gold watch syndrome', surviving five years before succumbing and see it as the beginning rather than the end, it should be (and is for most people) the start of a very happy era. The quality of life and accompanying fun increase markedly and remain so for a considerable number of years, in itself enhancing life expectancy.

Retirement, in its own right, can bring new and unusual hazards of an unexpected nature, and new ventures should be undertaken with caution. The experience of Rear Admiral Ian Robertson is a case in point. The admiral had lived a full life, packed with adventure accompanied by grave responsibility, which included being commanding officer of one of the Royal Navy's largest ships – the aircraft carrier HMS *Eagle* – a story to enthral in itself. As commanding officer, he was one of two officers holding a key to the ship's nuclear warheads. Power indeed, if only potential.

Now retired, preoccupied with golf, he felt inclined to broaden his interests and add a new dimension to his already extensive repertoire – cooking. Never inclined to do things by halves, he joined a cookery class, and soon felt a need to annexe the kitchen on a part-time basis. Broaching the subject to his wife, Barbara, a gentle but firm personality, he was taken aback when she was not wholly in accord with this uninvited intrusion into her terrain, as it did not fit in with her plans. Sizing up the situation, she suggested an alternative, and the admiral was despatched to an isolated hut at the bottom of the garden, with a small primus stove and a pan. The scene was set for an incident reminiscent of a scene featuring Alec Guinness in *Kind Hearts and Coronets*.

The admiral's cookery brief was simple enough: the instruction book was explicit. As the basis for a pudding, he read that he was to place three unopened tins of condensed milk into a saucepan, add water and bring it to the boil, before referring back for further instructions.

It was early afternoon, and the admiral, as befits his age, was in the habit of taking a postprandial nap. Having lit the primus, filled the pan with water, placed the tin of condensed milk in the water and put it on the primus, he sat down to await developments, which, in the event, were to prove dramatic. He would not have had long to wait for the water to boil, but his advancing years took their toll, and as he succumbed to his habitual catnap, which became slightly extended, the warning signs were lost on him. Indeed, the sound of water boiling only served as a soporific. In due course, the water boiled away, leaving the tin of condensed milk to heat up and assume, ironically, the characteristics of a potential warhead. The gathering storm continued to gather, and the climax came with dramatic suddenness.

Barbara, going about her business in the kitchen, was startled by a loud explosion, and looking into the garden was astonished to see enough steam coming out of the hut through a broken window to send a steam engine on its journey. Also, a bedraggled figure staggering forth from the hut, covered with liquid condensed milk, already congealing around the admiral's ample figure.

Fortunately no lasting damage was done, but the admiral now does a lot of cooking, under supervision, at the local cookery class, and is showing great promise. His friends much appreciate the results, and now he is occasionally allowed into Barbara's domain on parole! Remains of congealed caramel are still clinging to the walls of the hut, as testimony to yet another of the old seadog's adventures.

Second, unless struck down by terminal illness, there is a general feeling amongst those in their 7th and 8th decades of life that the quality of life could well continue to be most satisfactory up the end of the 8th decade (80), though a majority of people in their 60s had reservations as to what might happen thereafter and might well tend to become somewhat more problematic over the following 10 years.

Conversely, those around 80 remained much more optimistic about their own future, proving that they had not succumbed to ill health. This 'rolling optimism' is bolstered up by the fact that no matter how old you are, the statistical tables give encouragement by giving you a figure (in years) of how much longer you can expect to live – the nearest you are likely to get to being immortal!

Sadly, only a minority of the cases I have seen aged over 90 (and that includes the 799 in the list of cases I have summarised – see Figure XIII) unreservedly looked forward to another year of life. There were exceptions, like the centenarian who wrote in faultless script saying that the deterioration in reaching 100 made him feel 'seriously old'.

In conclusion, I can only say that it is not practical and might be most unwise to suggest a target age to live to. It is very much a personal matter, but for myself I have provisionally pencilled in 85, with the proviso that I retain dependable bowels, bladder, reasonable mobility, a sense of humour which *someone* might understand, and the right to change my mind at any stage, not excluding voluntary euthanasia.

I have discovered a further encouragement for endeavouring to extend my life: though I was terrified of women in my youth, I would hope that there will continue to be a sprinkling of sparkling ladies of my own vintage to spur me on!

I now refer to a 'budget date' of death which should not be confused with a 'target date'. A budget date of death is a date which can be determined at one's whim at any stage in life. Its purpose is not to state when one expects to die, but when one might die as a coldly calculated possibility, considering one's state of health and noting one's actuarial expectancy. Depending on this date (i.e., one's age) enables one to lay down some financial plans, such as divesting oneself of assets (for inheritance tax purposes), taking out life assurance (a gamble with the life assurance company), or even deciding whether to move to a smaller house.

Do You Want to Live a Little Longer?

A target date is more positive; how long I might live to (in contrast to a budget date – when might I die by). The budget date calls for financial provision, home accommodation, carers etc. I suspect that, like actuarial tables, this date will increase nearly, but not quite in line with one's actual age. The will to live is a potent factor!

One's age markedly influences one's attitude to death. In younger years few people give much thought to death, and it is left to the medical profession to suggest a number of precautionary steps to avoid illnesses, such as inoculations, giving up smoking, drinking less alcohol, and weight control.

In middling years most people take an increasing interest in death, and how to avoid, or at least postpone the ultimate event. They discover that there is quite a lot that one can do to this end, of which giving up smoking, the largest cause of premature death, is but one step, though arguably the most important one. At about the same time (in middle age), people become increasingly aware that some ways of exiting this life are preferable to others, though the main aim, at least until about age 70, is to avoid the happening in any form! At all stages so far, people are prepared to go to considerable pains and lengths to circumvent life-threatening illnesses, even submitting to sophisticated and painful surgical procedures (coronary by-pass surgery is a good example).

After about the age of 70, a progressive change starts influencing one's 'death philosophy'. The death vehicle remains very important; 75% of people over 70 are more concerned as to how they are going to die rather than when. It is important to bear in mind that, at 70, you may either be lucky, or have adapted a sensible lifestyle which has kept you alive and relatively free from gross discomforts.

You now need to review your health philosophy. Having avoided some lethal illnesses earlier (terminal, but not necessarily unpleasant otherwise, a coronary for example), you have now survived to become a candidate for another mode of death which may not be acceptable when it confronts you.

The practical implication is that, to take one example, there has been an increase of 27% in the diagnoses of cancer in women, and 20% in men between 1979 and 1990; the former figure has been caused by the increase in smoking by women.

I therefore commend a philosophy for your consideration which might well be termed the 'roulette philosophy'. You have accumulated considerable 'survival winnings' (you are now over 70), and might well feel that you can relax on some of those factors which have enabled you to survive so long. A number of illnesses, not all of them life-threatening, are lining up to stake a claim to your body and mind. The time has come to regard the remainder of your years as a gamble, for that is what life is, the more so the older one gets. Therefore, approach the remaining years rather like a game of *vingt-et-un*, where one examines one's cards and makes a decision either to 'stick' or 'twist'. If you twist (perhaps major surgery) you might be over bold and not recover from a complex surgical operation, or ultra-cautious by declining treatment, resulting in early death (*vingt-et-un's* equivalent of sticking). Alternatively, by declining treatment you might well be extending your life because the medical condition didn't prove to be so fatally flawed as was feared.

One example of sticking was Howard Hughes, the American aircraft designer, who elected to stick by rigorously isolating himself from any form of contact with the outside world, morbidly fearful of infection. As a result he led a miserable life and died from a non-infectious disease at a comparatively early age.

To sum it up:

a) Take note of the identifiable life-threatening habits throughout the middle years, and live in a way that avoids them.

b) After 70, progressively ease up and enjoy what is available and within one's capabilities. Treat yourself, for 'a little of what you fancy does you good'.

c) After the mid-70s or so, consider very carefully the merits of whether to submit to 'heroic' surgical interference offered as 'life-saving', when, by so doing, one might be condemned to a much worse end than might ensue from adopting a policy of 'masterly inactivity' leavened with a little palliative treatment and tender loving care (TLC).

Cradle to Grave

In 1944, whilst still a medical student, I was fortunate enough to meet Sir William Beveridge (later Lord Beveridge) who hoped to become an MP as the Liberal candidate for Hexham – a widely spread parliamentary constituency in the North of England. I was invited to spend the day with Sir William and Lady Beveridge as they toured Northumberland. The Beveridge plan had just been published, and, not unnaturally, Sir William spent a good part of the day talking with justifiable pride about his panacea for making health available without charge to everybody. I recall contemplating two things which concerned me even as a young man:

1) How to provide infinite medical care to an already forecasted ageing population from finite resources, at a time when diagnostic procedures and subsequent treatment were scheduled to become increasingly sophisticated and expensive. Even then it was evident that 'rationing' of treatment would make the concept difficult to fund, and so it has proved to be.

The shortfall between demand for medical resources and their provision has been exacerbated by a factor which was not anticipated in the Beveridge Report, namely the massive increase in the numbers of immigrants entering the United Kingdom. For example, citizens of Asian extraction have, for reasons which have not been explained, an above average incidence of renal failure, leading to unusually heavy demands for kidney transplants. Ethnic minorities also suffer from an above average incidence of tuberculosis; there is also a higher than usual incidence of mental breakdown amongst immigrants.

There was already talk about the necessity of managers who would run this Health Service with the aim of allowing doctors to get on with their primary task of treating patients. My fear was that it would be the managers who would make decisions on who would be rationed! And so it has come to be.

2) It was clear from Sir Willliam's ideological approach that the medical profession would have to submit to the control of politicians (themselves transient, and primarily concerned with their own short-term political health). Thus I believed then and still do, that the profession was doomed to lose control, not only of its own destiny, but also to a large extent of its patients' best interests.

What I learned that day determined my own future; I resolved not to join the National Health Service, and subsequently joined the Royal Navy, a step I never regretted.

It would be wrong to leave the subject there, for, though events have largely justified that decision, for myself it must be put on record that there is one aspect of the NHS that cannot be equalled, and that is accident and emergency care, for here doctors are allowed to do what seems to be in the best interest of the patient, without being directed by managers.

It was with these thoughts in my mind that, in May 1994, I read about a case which well illustrated the second of my fears. It concerned a 72-year-old man who suffered from osteoarthritis and had been in the habit of receiving physiotherapy at his local hospital. What appeared to be a satisfactory arrangement was brought to an abrupt halt when the authorities discovered the patient's age, and ordered him to be transferred to a nearby geriatric hospital. Unfortunately there were no facilities for physiotherapy at the geriatric hospital and the treatment came to a stop.

I wrote a letter to *The Daily Telegraph* on the subject (see Appendix III). As a result, I received dozens of letters direct to my home, in spite of the limited address given. They included:

1) One from a centenarian, typed by himself and signed in perfect script, strongly resenting being categorised by the phrase 'old person', the media being particularly guilty in this regard, or, worse still, as a 'pensioner'. On reaching 100, he was startled at the sudden changes that suddenly overtook him, though he boasted that he was still able to look after himself, his flat, and to shop and cook for himself fully independently. He remembers the Boxer Rebellion, has written 18 books, been a scriptwriter in Hollywood, still supervises the production of his plays in Europe, and 'travels regularly'. He attributes his longevity to:

> *In this dark world of sin and strife.*
> *How have I lived so long?*
> *A Godly, righteous and sober life.*
> *With wine, women and song.*

If slightly contradictory, one must make some allowances. (His name is E.G. Cousins, and he lives in Devon).

2) A man (writing from Spain) who had founded a public company (Arndale Developments) and had been angered when he was retired at 65. He emigrated to Spain and formed a similar company (Arndale Centres Espagna) and, as chairman, at the age of 90 still guides the company with a considerable and continuing programme of work, 'keeping up the standards'.

3) Another, who reapplied for his driving licence at 103, was not only relieved when it arrived, but delighted to get a reduced quote from his insurers for his car, although it is not clear on what grounds.

4) An aggrieved son who was astonished when his 90-year-old father decided to emigrate by himself to South Africa; he returned to England (unaccompanied) to play the organ at his great-niece's wedding before returning 'home' to South Africa.

5) An octogenarian who stroked an octogenarian 'four' over the course at Henley-on-Thames.

6) A seventy-eight-year youngster who plays 3 sets of tennis (with others of similar age) every Saturday in the year.

7)   Many others from varied walks of life, including a lollipop man.

8)   And also a telephone call from a 76-year-old chief flying instructor at North Weald.   Noting his age, I unwisely enquired whether he was a 'non-playing captain', only to receive a flea in my ear.   I was very firmly told, "Indeed not; I personally conduct every final flying test on every pupil in this club."   All I could say was, "Yes, sir!"

Medical Insurance.

This is a highly charged political area.   The choice lies anywhere between full private cover to putting aside an amount equivalent to the insurance premium and so building up a reserve to enable one to purchase private treatment should the necessity arise.   Like most insurance, it is a gamble, assuming that one requires private treatment anyway.   It would seem rational to assess one's chances of requiring expensive treatment before the average person, and if in your favour, accumulate a 'sinking fund' up to a certain age, say 65, and then commence insurance cover, meanwhile spending the sinking fund on a very good holiday, thus extending one's life expectancy anyway!

The 'Silent Telephone' Syndrome.

This is the retirement equivalent of the 'empty cot syndrome' affecting mothers when their fledglings leave home.

The sad overtones from all the letters I received in response to my letter in *The Daily Telegraph* was that they were all from people over 75, and one could also sense that they felt, in spite of their continuing achievements, 'discouraged by society from making a meaningful contribution'.

There is a rational explanation for these valuable and worthy elder citizens feeling that they are 'not wanted'; that is a negative feeling.   It is not that they are no longer wanted so much as no longer required.

Increasingly in the age of information technology it is not what man knows, but, to quote that old saw, it is who he knows, or, to bring it up to date, how much he knows, and more importantly where the information is to be found.   As less and less real knowledge is available today, people increasingly resort to buzz words like 'data bank' or 'the media', and people with access to 'an ear' (radio), the Press or the media in general are listened to. It doesn't matter whether they talk sense or not; a 'view' is put across, for the media is power today.

To be still working implies power and 'access' to corridors of power in their various forms. One is useful or, to be exact, has a use. Having a use implies access to money, and so back to argentosis with all its attendant complications such as being practised in being economical with the truth, and all that follows in the wake of such standards.

With retirement, the mantle (for that is all being employed means) falls away, and behold, the Emperor has no clothes and no mystique with it. Then the telephone stops ringing, not suddenly but progressively, unnoticed at first. Telephone silence comes on insidiously and with it a falling-off of contacts and up-to-date useful information. It is from such matters that retired people begin to feel discouraged and ultimately not wanted.

It is with sadness that, from my own observation, those over 70 tend to be ignored in committee meetings where there exists an age differential of more that 10–15 years between the 'oldie' and the rest.

Retirement is the most difficult career which faces anybody, and calls for preparation. Many feel that it is a release from persecution or even slavery, but having become a near-lifetime routine the event of catching the train is surprisingly missed. Some face the release as a heaven-sent opportunity to catch up on all those little tasks, but there is a limit to how many times the decorating can be done, the garden dug, or *The Times* crossword finished (the 5-year gold watch death syndrome). Most people come to terms with retirement as such, simply taking 30% longer to complete a task (if it hadn't already happened before retirement), which is an ominous sign. Some take up serious golf or find other congenial ways to occupy the days. Others attempt to pursue long-awaited joys such as serious sailing, mountaineering, even skiing, only to find that they have left it too late for their brittle joints to cope.

For a minority without a hobby or time-consuming interest, time hangs heavily, and they begin to notice that the telephone doesn't ring quite so often, leading to an almost paranoid suspicion that they are being left out. Those who have retired from a bustling, important appointment wonder why their opinion is no longer sought, on something, anything, not appreciating that it was not their wisdom which had been sought but information of some sort purely related to their position, a position now occupied by another.

Inevitably, friendships were forged during working lives, but sadly only a minority of such 'friendships' are likely to survive once the business catalyst is severed.

Similarly, the daily post diminishes, except for junk mail, and it requires a lot of family understanding to help the newly retired member of society to adjust, in many cases a proffering of sympathy.

Given patience, this new-found spare time can be turned to considerable advantage; unrealised and untapped mental capabilities can be developed and a vast majority of newly retired people adjust well in welcoming the new challenge. Those who are able to turn their back on the past without regret appear to derive the biggest pleasure from their new-found leisure, and though they may seem 'dated' in their outlook by the younger generation, there is enormous pleasure and satisfaction to be had during retirement.

Taking up writing remains an ever-present option, irrespective of age, and one that is stimulating, as it calls for constant reading, which is the equivalent of keeping the door open to the world.

But that phone? It will still not ring quite so often as it did pre-retirement! Maybe there is some rewarding research to be done for a Ph.D. thesis on: 'The correlation between disability, older years, and telephone usage'.

Bear in mind that retirement hobbies need careful selection.

It has been suggested that sex discrimination extends into the older years. One Kit Pyman investigated and found that, in spite of women living longer than their male counterparts, and therefore being greater in number, they featured much less in some 12 magazines which she researched; when they did, usually in pictures, it was as if by accident, and women rarely featured in the text or editorial.

I became slightly sceptical and Kit went on to observe that when pictures of older men were featured they invariably had 'gorgeous blondes on their arms'. She offered an explanation: perhaps the older woman has a bad image in the public mind, tending to be featured as mother-in-law, dowager, bag lady (*Oxford English Dictionary*: 'slightly derogatory; a woman, esp. regarded as unattractive, unpleasant: baggy folds under the eyes'), overweight granny, or tottering OAP in need of charity.

Do you think that there could be an explanation here for why males chuck their hand in and die some five years before their females? No, a more likely explanation for Kit's dismay about the older woman not featuring is that even now women simply do not feature even as younger persons in the open market as much as men, and this simply continues as a prejudice into the older years.

Men will get their comeuppance before long, I believe. For example, have you noticed the increasing number of female bus drivers, and how much smoother a ride they give compared with their male counterparts?

Chapter Eleven
The Six Ages of Man

The six ages of man: though life expectancy has not lengthened materially in recent years there has been a cohort of 'ageing' people advancing into later years. This, coupled with vastly increasing facilities enabling these 'older' people to continue participating in a variety of activities such as travel, information, intellectual pursuits and so on, means that it is no longer appropriate or even accurate to talk about life's 'three score years and ten'. Moreover, the hypothetical 'generation gap' has narrowed to a point where it is barely discernible, and when it is, the older person is labelled as 'stuffy' or 'behind the times' and misses fun accordingly.

To keep abreast of changing circumstances, it seems appropriate to review the 'ages of man', and there would now seem to be six ages with subtle but distinct differences (see Figure IX).

The attribute 'wisdom' is one characteristic which can only stem from experience and is therefore present only in older people. Conversely, not all older people become wise, so a mixture of watching, listening and intelligence is also required; even those with experience and skill are not necessarily wise.

Wisdom is at the opposite end of the intelligence spectrum to computer knowledge. It is something which cannot be taught, and therefore cannot be 'learnt' in the academic sense of the word.

For those older persons who possess wisdom, their counsel, if sought, can be invaluable. The modern trend to retire persons early, often against their inclination, is to be deplored, throwing a disproportionate and unnecessary burden on the 'earning' section of the community.

Those people categorised as elderly (65–85) constitute a source of wisdom greater than all the reference libraries put together, but, unlike the libraries, their values are rarely utilised.

FIGURE IX: THE SIX AGES OF MAN

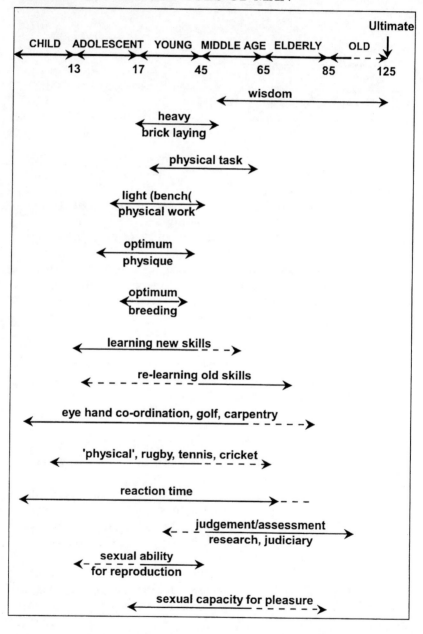

Most of the factors in the diagrams are self-explanatory, save for one. This one commands a disproportionate share of the nation's gross national product; it is the subject of sex and all that follows in its wake.

Sexual Prowess:

This has been divided into two categories: 'sexual ability' and 'sexual capability'.

a) Sexual Ability. This term is used in a purely biological or reproductive context, as in cattle breeding. This may sound crude, but is simply pragmatic, for if the best strains are to be used to produce the future human race, breeding should be from the best strains and whilst the breeders are at peak performance. But decreasing sperm mobility may be yet another potential threat to propagating the human race.

These are shades of *Brave New World* (do I hear 'cloning'?) and unlikely to come about, but the present system is not working (one in three marriages ending in divorce) and is causing untold misery both to parents and children alike, not to mention grandparents.

Research has not yet demonstrated to what extent society is threatened by the growth in marital breakdown and the increasing number of single parent families, but it cannot be satisfactory. The human species itself may even be threatened. Perhaps divorce is itself a symptom of some underlying social or intellectual sickness in society. Research is particularly lacking on these points. Perhaps research is not necessary, for perhaps it is blatantly obvious.

But to take one general point: is the species (modern man) happy? Animals cease to breed if they are not content or are subject to extreme privation. By this definition the evidence would seem to signal that all is well, but that would be to fly in the face of the evidence. It must be viewed from another aspect.

There would appear to be a strong correlation between broken homes, disturbances in family life and crime, even the sheer 'cussedness' so common today. Though the recorded incidence of marital break-up is known, it is not known how much further submerged unhappiness and discord exists that was not actually broken in statistical records.

Is it possible that the wide variety of sexual deviations practised today may be a symptomatic by-product of the stresses experienced in modern life?

b) Sexual Capability. This like wisdom would appear to come later in life when the 'instant sex' desires have abated somewhat, become less blatant and are discussed more rationally and openly. For those fortunate enough to have found capability as a part of a loving relationship, energies previously dissipated in the sexual fantasy world are now available to be deployed elsewhere in other more constructive pursuits.

Perhaps society is in the revolutionary process of discovering that there are two separate interpretations of the sexual habit, and when this has been written into the 'code of life' (and accepted by the Church), civilisation might become secure and progressive once more. Perhaps the Church should abandon its conception of 'marriage for life', and substitute, if only tacitly, two distinct marital ceremonies: one for the purpose of breeding and one for 'companionship', the latter being the more stable. There could be a fundamental change in the Church's attitude to marriage and divorce, enabling second marriages to take place within the Church, but fully recognising them as forms of marriage. Reciprocally, as well as 'bringing the Church to the people', it might even 'bring the people to the Church'.

Perhaps that old British standby, a Royal Commission, should be set up to examine the whole matter.

Medicine might be called upon to recognise sexual prowess as a measurable entity like a blood count or thyroid activity, and contained till it can be productively utilised, like any similar endocrine activity. Too much (especially if joined with promiscuity) can be health-threatening, embarrassing, and even dangerous if not contained. To define sexual prowess might not be appropriate, but, to embrace a Rolls Royce approach when describing the power of their car engines, the 'description sufficient for the purpose' might be apt!

FIGURE X: AGE AND SKILL

A) MANUAL CO-ORDINATION – Minimal intellectual input e.g. labouring

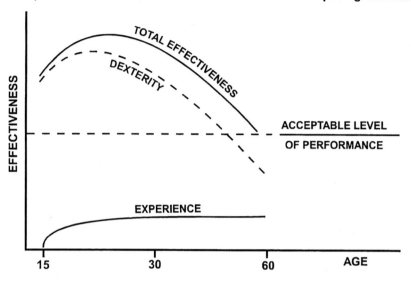

B) PROPRIOCEPTIVE ABILITIES – 'Hand-eyes' co-ordination, ball games

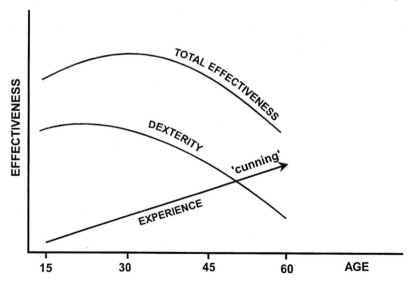

FIGURE XI: COMPUTER SKILL

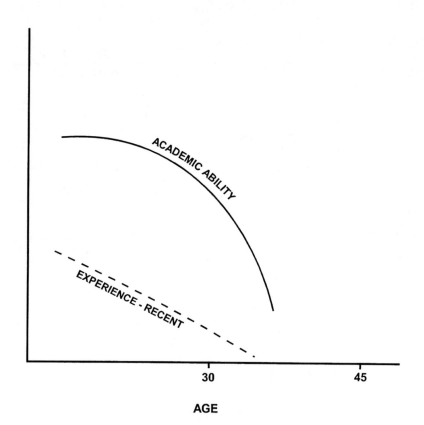

Figure X (A) illustrates the relationship between age, assuming normal health, and a demanding physical task; experience plays a little part in the effectiveness, and the level at which acceptability plays a part revolves around and is dependent upon the level at which 'reward for the job' is pitched. To a large extent this is influenced by union pressure. This is finite, and trade unions have a heavy responsibility as to whether their members continue to be employed or not, for if unions press for ever-increasing wages, the 'acceptable level of performance' line will progressively move upwards and result in members becoming unemployable. See also Figure IV on page 75.

Figure X (B) relates to proprioceptive abilities: the hand-eye coordination involved in ball games like golf, tennis, cricket and squash. Providing such pursuits are indulged in for pleasure rather than for reward (see above), then, helped with the progressive replacement of skill by 'cunning' (experience) such pursuits can be followed to a considerable age.

By contrast to intellectual or physically demanding pursuits computer skills (see Figure XI) are in a different class; not really demanding in terms of scholastic ability, the science of computers has moved at an astonishingly fast pace, so that computer intelligence is increasingly replacing human intelligence. The latter is strong in decision taking, a distinct disadvantage in computer working, which is strong on logic and numeracy. A high but specialised intellectual skill is required at the creative stage in computer design, but only moderate intelligence is required to operate computers.

Computers are developing at such a pace that experience obtained on one 'family' of computers soon becomes obsolete and transient in value and can even be a handicap when applied to a new generation of computers. Thus middle-aged people can be quite baffled and frustrated (another form of stress!) if confronted by a comparatively simple computer task, such as setting a video programme, even though it is logical and simple, as opposed to simple logical minds brought up in the 'new age', i.e., the computer age.

Computers Don't Cry – They're Clinical

Within living memory of approximately 50% of today's Western world population, more 'progress' has been made than has taken place since the evolution of man's ability to communicate by speech (100,000 years ago).

This advancement, or 'progress', has, until the last 40 years or so, been spread fairly evenly, right across the path of man's discoveries, and so has advanced the cause of 'civilisation' as a whole entity.

During the last 40 years, however, this progress has partly, or wholly in some instances, been as the result of the direct, or indirect evolution of the microchip, which has changed, and continues to change the very life pattern of the human species. By so doing, it is now the most singularly important factor threatening *Homo sapiens'* continuing existence on planet Earth, and with it, that of many other species in the 6th Mass Extinction (see Chapter Two).

The benefits, and temptations from becoming increasingly dependent on chips are as insidious and habit-forming as drugs, as the more the human race comes to depend on them, the more demands are made for 'more', whilst simultaneously eroding man's independence.

To the older person it seems strange how dependent a young shop assistant appears to be on an 'adding machine' when calculating the change required when buying a newspaper.

There can be but one end to this 'progress' – when all individuals are programmed by computers, themselves programmed by a minority master race, increasingly rarefied in number, having replaced the previous master race – for example, accountants – having eliminated lower grade skills in the process.

Let us examine two widely differing disciplines which are already very much influenced, if not dominated by computers – both of which I have been considerably involved in.

Medicine

Historically, this profession has been an 'art', backed up by help from 'science' when called upon. 'Faith' (not to be confused with 'faith healing'), but rather in the nature of 'trust' or 'confidence', has been an essential part of the process of therapeutic healing. This brings into play an essential ingredient in the relationship – tactility, in itself as important a part of the diagnostic content as is the establishment of confidence.

The proper establishment of this basis is time intensive, and cannot be rushed. Demands for productivity would be self-defeating, for time spent in examining – be it 'hands on', 'eyes on' or simply 'listening to' is rarely wasted – indeed, it is the cornerstone of good clinical medicine.

The time-honoured greeting 'How are you?' is being replaced by 'What is the matter with you?' (surely the doctor's task to find out!), and increasingly by a tendency to circumvent all unnecessary questions with a request for a sample of some bodily fluid or other, accompanied by a 'deferred judgement' pending the result, and yet a further appointment.

Home calls – in themselves an important part of the diagnostic procedure on certain occasions – have been virtually eliminated, except for the purpose of signing a death certificate – though at least such documents are not yet post-dated!

One feels that the days of multiple-choice questionnaires, do-it-yourself diagnoses and e-mail evaluations may not be far off.

Society gets the medical service it chooses, and deserves, and a health service dominated by politicians, or politically correct administrators will not have the users in society's best interests at heart, for their policies will be dominated by their treasury masters, and inevitably the quality of care will deteriorate.

A medical qualification may not be ideal for drawing up a financial budget, but if adequate health care standards are to be achieved, commensurate with what funds are available, then the development of those funds are better left to be allocated by those appropriately qualified in medical matters, rather than by lay 'medical' administrators.

Ominously, the ultimate destiny of medical treatment is not wholly currently in medical hands. If bureaucracy is deemed essential, there could be a case for abbreviating the current six-year medical course, and establishing a 'fast track' to a restricted medical qualification, and associated limited clinical responsibility – much as can be found in a co-pilot's duties in commercial airline practice.

Aviation

Flying and pilots can still conjure up a picture of Biggles, equipped with goggles; and an air of glamour, if not prestige is discernible around any airport – though this image is fading fast, and anyone harbouring it today is likely to have aspirations akin to 'train-spotting'. The more realistic happening, and the nearest one might come to spotting such a person, is the glimpse of a figure in dark uniform, with gold stripes on his (or increasingly her) nonchalantly unbuttoned uniform, inconspicuously wandering across the concourse – almost 'depersonalised', having the appearance, for all they might be, of a computer operator – and indeed, that is what they are, bearing little resemblance to the old-style aviators, for much of their professional skill has been considerably subjugated to the microchip's influence.

As young people have lost the ability to do simple arithmetic to the world of adding machines, so rudimentary flying skills are practised less (and therefore become less practised), being taken over by computers. Such computers may function in a direct mode, as in any part of the aircraft's extended flight envelope from the moment of take-off to the moment of touchdown, or in an indirect mode, as in a simulator on the ground. The latter, whilst fulfilling a valuable, indeed essential training or examinational role, can only simulate the real situation, and is therefore 'ersatz'.

As progress continues, enabling microchips to erode and eventually replace human skills with a higher degree of precision, an important, even dangerous characteristic of computers is emerging – a form of self-destruction.

At the present, computers follow a predetermined programme, are unable to react to errors which have inadvertently been fed into their programme, nor initiate a change of plan, which has not been 'programmed', in order to rectify a deteriorating situation.

Such a situation occurred when an Airbus was demonstrating a low-level, low--speed 'fly-past' to spectators in France. The aircraft was trimmed into the landing configuration (undercarriage flaps down etc.), and the computer prepared the aircraft to land on a non-existent runway. In spite of the pilot's best endeavours to take over the worsening situation, the autopilot would have none of it, and the aircraft crashed. An excellent demonstration – up to that point!

Such is the background to the story that, in a very advanced computer-dominated aircraft, there would be only one person on the flight deck – the pilot, but there would also be a Rottweiler. Stripped of any real responsibility, the sole task of the pilot would be to keep the Rottweiler content – feeding him etc. The purpose of the

Rottweiler would be to prevent the pilot from touching any of the controls!

Historically, as aircraft developed and the parameters of aviation were explored – height, speed etc. – many accidents, often fatal, happened. Invariably, the causes were mechanical failures, in one form or another, as the frontiers of flying were probed.

Eventually, the parameters within which conventional aircraft were to operate were laid down, and engineering progress made flying safer. Not so for the humans flying sophisticated (military) machines, however, who are, unlike the aircraft, incapable of 'being developed', but have to rely upon artificial means of protection from the hostile environment (reduced atmospheric pressure, heavy G-forces etc.), and match up to increased mental demands made upon them.

It is not surprising, therefore, that now, although flying has become very much safer, the accidents that do happen are invariably caused by human error, thus increasing the cry for more help from computers. This becomes a vicious circle, for the more help from computers, the less there is for a pilot to do during an extended flight, so that boredom and consequent fatigue set in, with a yet lower performance levels from the pilots.

Help could be at hand though. With the development of telemetry, and a high degree of reliability, and pending full automation replacing aircrew, there is no reason why aircraft should not be landed by a pilot sitting in a simulator on the ground– locked to the approaching aircraft via telemetering equipment, and control being executed some 100 miles (say) before touchdown. Thus, all aircraft leaving, and destined for an airport, would be directly controlled by a team of specialist pilots, sitting together at the destination airport, who would be in constant practice at landing.

There would be several advantages from such a development:

a)   The skill required for landing would always be immediately available in practised hands, and local conditions intimately understood.

b)   The on-board pilot would be released to look after the interests of the passengers, socialising, as happens in passenger ships, and restoring the personal touch that once existed. Boredom would be a thing of the past.

c)   The captain's secondary role would be to stand by to cope with any untoward emergency, or diversion to other destinations.   To maximise efficiency, there would be interchange at regular intervals between the on-board captain, and the effective pilot on the ground, thus ensuring that all roles were kept at operational effectiveness.

Policing Computers

Because computers are unable to recognise their own failings, and will obey any recognised command, they are fully exposed to exploitation by 'unauthorised' criminals, and become accomplices in fraud on an unprecedented scale.   To prevent this, an up-dated equivalent of the Dickensian character who ticked every ledger entry with a quill pen is required.   This should lie within the skills of a new make of computer!

The main threat to civilisation is not, however, on account of potential fraud – though this is very real.   It is the removal of the opportunity for humans to carry out simple tasks, and the isolation of individuals from one another in the meeting place.

This is already taking place – for example, the high street meeting place has been replaced by huge food stores, with their impersonal atmospheres, and the balance of human emotions and relations has become disturbed.   The resultant deprivation may well be a factor in some of the present social malpractices evident today – such as road rage.

Intellectual Skills

One of the characteristics of advancing years is that change is not readily accepted, for it implies an effort to accommodate change (see Chapter Nine).   For this reason, it requires an effort to make decisions, unless to retain the *status quo*, and thus any call to make any decision is increasingly avoided, for changes are anathema to advancing years.

To retain the benefit of the intrinsic wisdom of the older executive therefore, he should be retained as an adviser only.   A further refinement of this belief is that the same restriction applies to the non-executive director, for he too will prefer to support the *status quo*.   Perhaps there is a case for the creation of a new 'non-voting,

FIGURE XII: INTELLECTUAL SKILLS

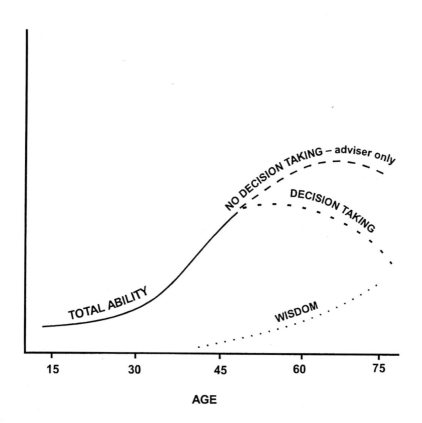

non-executive director' or, to put it simply, an 'advisory director'. The elderly are particularly suited to this role. (See Figure XII.)

Effect Of Age On Re-Learning Skills.

If you don't want to lose it USE it

Modern Saying

It is a common belief that one never forgets how to ride a bicycle. This is a myth; one does forget, sometimes with disastrous results.

Chapter Twelve
Behind the Lace Curtains

In repeatedly returning to the quest about the mysteries of death, it was becoming increasingly clear that the whole subject was as impenetrable as the mysteries of the universe itself, and that all that could be done was to send probes into the subject and listen to people who had been near to death themselves or who had been, or were currently, in close contact with someone in the last phases of life.

Even that revealed relatively little, for although, like the universe, it was clear to see, it was difficult to comprehend; both could be pointed at, but without certainty as to the reality. So to begin with, I concluded that the examination of a body after death was of little more use than examining the skin of a snake after its owner had shed it. It might reveal something about the former inhabitant, the mode of death or even the circumstances, but little or nothing about what death was in the abstract sense.

In the absence of firm evidence from the crucible of death, it is easy to understand how religion has been able to establish a diktat over the living; whatever might be said, providing it is said with conviction, could not be challenged, at least not on grounds of fact!

A research campaign was called for to investigate. The possibility of studying and interviewing a considerable number of people during the final few days or weeks of their lives was not immediately practical; it would be confining as well as probably being morbid, depressing, and intrusive.

The next most practical thing might be to see people who were in the autumn of their lives, who, though not overshadowed by the thought of an imminent demise, might well be aware that it would happen sometime in the not too far distant future. An added attraction was that already it seemed to me that the 'elderly' were getting a good deal more enjoyment and satisfaction than many younger people from the troubled society in which we struggle, and which appears to thrust problems of such magnitude upon us that misery seems to abound. No wonder that retired people derive such enjoyment when released from work, in spite of gathering disabilities. They seem to be contributing so much more to life's rich tapestry, and, like an ageing bottle of good claret, though covered in dust, with the label partly obscured, hold a great deal more to offer if patiently savoured.

There was another personally compelling reason for conducting the extended research programme amongst the elderly population. At that time it would not be long before I too would be manoeuvring into the little-known waters of the eighth decade, and thoughts of retirement were beginning to formulate; it was becoming increasingly clear that retirement would be a challenge and probably the most difficult yet important 'career' of one's life. Muff it, and soon, from my observations of others, it would be a case of 'Come in, no. 9, time's up'. I reckon that I had bought myself some extended time by at least paying some attention to my earlier lifestyle (eating, some exercise, avoiding becoming too involved with the domestic routine), but then one couldn't altogether rely upon the validity of the extension, rather like buying an airline ticket from a little-known bucket shop (though the nature of the destinations are different!).

Age has a habit of creeping up upon one, though with some possibly unwelcome surprises. The more retired people whom I saw, the more daunting the prospect of retirement became. How should one set about it? Were there any courses that one might attend? The best thing to do would seem to be to go and learn from those who had already retired, and learn from their successes and failures.

In the event, fate took me by the hand and the appropriate door opened.

I read in the *British Medical Journal* about how the Health and Safety at Work Act was approved by all political parties, and that the medical 'back-up' was to be expanded and revamped and to be called the Employment Medical Advisory Service (EMAS). The plan was to make EMAS largely independent of, but advisory to, the Health and Safety Executive, itself the 'working' arm of the Health and Safety Commission. The whole scheme seemed over-ambitious, but a substantial recruiting drive for medical officers, with or without industrial medical experience, had been launched. More important to me, they needed a number of part-time doctors, which suited me as I preferred to have a number of part-time occupations, thus retaining some control over what I chose to do week by week.

So I resumed my medical career as a part-time medical officer in the Employment Medical Advisory Service of the Health and Safety Executive, in the county of Wiltshire, and spent my remaining time doing medical rehabilitation, as well as reports for the Department of Health and Social Security on applicants for Attendance Allowance and Mobility Allowance. This covered some 22 years from 1970 to 1992.

Between 1970 and 1992, a total of 10,209 patients were seen by me, mostly in connection with applications for Attendance Allowance, a government cash allowance granted to those persons deemed to meet strictly laid-down conditions and requiring assistance in connection with their bodily needs. The vast majority of these cases were seen in their own homes, a procedure which has many advantages and is as different to seeing a patient in a formal surgery environment as seeing animals in the wild compared with a zoo. The average examination lasted one and a quarter hours, with a maximum of three hours, the shortest a few minutes, the latter being curtailed by the threat of an assault by the patient!

Location

The 10,209 cases were seen over a wide and varied area from the Midlands to the South coast of England, as well as in Central London. This included the counties of the West Midlands, Worcestershire and Herefordshire, Warwickshire, Oxfordshire, Gloucestershire, Wiltshire, Dorset and Hampshire, and Middlesex, ten counties in all.

Excluding the cases seen in London, approximately half the cases were visited in rural areas and the remainder in urban areas.

The cases are summarised in Figure XIII, below.

FIGURE XIII

AGE (90+)	799 (7.8%)
ARTHRITIS	753 (7.4%)
CANCER (LUNG & BREAST = 50% +)[1]	692 (6.8%)
CVA	691 (6.8%)
DEMENTIA	667 (6.6%)
OSTEOARTHRITIS FRACTURES	552 (5.4%)
PATIENTS WITH LEARNING DISABILITIES	410 (4%)
CONGENITAL JOINT DISEASE REPLACEMENTS	344 (3.4%)
COAD	303 (3%)
PARKINSON'S DISEASE	296 (2.9%)
CIRCULATORY DISORDERS	279 (2.7%)
CARDIAC	277 (2.7%)
PSYCHOSES	267 (2.6%)
ATHEROSCLEROSIS	219 (2.2%)
AMPUTEE (LL)	211 (2.1%)
MS	189 (1.9%)
RTA	182 (1.85%)
DIABETES	152 (1.5%)
BLIND	140 (1.4%)
DOWN'S SYNDROME	138 (1.4%)
ANGINA	114 (1.1%)
SPASTIC DIPLEGIA	113 (1.1%)
MISCELLANEOUS (I) < 5 CASES PER DIAGNOSIS	601 (5.9 %)
MISCELLANEOUS (II) > 5 CASES PER DIAGNOSIS	⇨1461 (14.3%)
MISCELLANEOUS (III) NO DIAGNOSIS	359 (3.5%)

---

[1] Cancer affects one person in three at some point in their lives.

Statistics Relating to Figure XIII

Miscellaneous (ii) includes:

Epilepsy	91 (0.9%)
Brain tumour	84 (0.8%)
Sub-arachnoid haemorrhage	64 (0.4%)
Motor neurone disease	58 (0.6%)
Polio	35 (0.4%)
AIDS	49 (0.5%)
TB	29 (0.3%)
Alcohol dependence	29 (0.3%)
Endocrinology-related	20 (0.2%)
'Grief'	17 (0.2%)

Total cases seen: 10, 209

Analysis

More than 600 different diagnoses were made, covering a wide variety of afflictions. Not all cases were imminently terminal, although a high proportion of patients had a very limited expectation of life.

Certain illnesses do not feature in the table, as the terms of reference for seeing patients did not cover short-term illnesses such as most acute infections, those causing sudden death, fatal coronaries, less severe injuries resulting from road traffic accidents, suicides, ruptured blood vessels, or certain acute catastrophes (although victims surviving such catastrophes might still feature).

Similarly, at 1.5% of the cases seen, the number of diabetes-related disabilities, which include amputations, comas, blindness, secondary infections, to mention but a few, is not representative of the incidence of diabetes as a whole. Including those not dependent on insulin, diabetes mellitus – to give it its full title – affects 6% of the population at large. This is not to minimise the seriousness of diabetes, but is a good example of how sensible care and lifestyle can control even a potentially dangerous disease.

Approximately one quarter of *all* diagnoses were smoking-related, and the role of smoking in illness generally has been confirmed in other studies on smoking and health.

One overall trend in the long-term shift from bacteria-orientated diseases to 'structural' or traumatic diseases was confirmed.

A refreshing fact is that 'old age' heads the list of 'diagnoses' (nearly 8% of all cases seen). For the purpose of this particular study, 'old age' was identified as a diagnosis if the patient had reached 90 or more, and, although few of such cases were without symptoms of some incapacitating complaint or other, they were judged to be capable of living a more or less independent life. However, a significant number in this category tended to say that they had 'just about had enough', intimating that, for a variety of reasons, the quality of life had deteriorated to a level where their well-being was seriously affected. What they would have said if the 'way out' had been available I do not know.

Apart from 'age' (7.8%), the next four commonest diseases were arthritis (i.e. general, rather that osteoarthritis which affects a specific joint), cancer, stroke, and dementia made up over a quarter of the cases (27.6%), so this gives some indication of what lies in store if other life-threatening afflictions are side-stepped earlier in life.

Technique

To be effective, the confidence of the patient had to be gained as quickly as possible; as one female patient said, "I don't think doctors realise how terrifying it is to expect, and await, a call from a stranger, whom they haven't met; not knowing what form or extent of examination one is going to be given – and all because one has applied for a small sum of money in order to go on living in one's own home."

Another patient, echoing these sentiments, told me, "I dread consulting a doctor. Much prefer going to the dentist – at least I know which orifice is going to be explored."

The Bird

It was soon evident that people who have a chronic or even a drawn-out terminal illness invariably keep a pet of some sort, of which the commonest are dogs, or cats, followed by fish or birds. The trait may well be symptomatic of loneliness associated with the elderly and living alone. Close bonds of mutual trust are forged between these living creatures and their owners, and the animals seem to take on some of the characteristics of guide dogs and become fiercely possessive. One way I found of gaining the trust of the patient was to spend approximately five minutes concentrating on the animal, usually a dog. During this time, and the animals quickly assess whether you are 'visitor friendly', the owner watches intently to see how you are assessed. If one was accepted, which was invariably the case, then the acceptance extended to the patient, and at once opened up the atmosphere to a degree of warmth which made life easier for all concerned.

On occasions, on ringing the doorbell one could hear sounds of scuffling, interspersed with the odd whimper or sharp word, whilst the animal was confined out of sight. This was something I always countermanded, releasing the animal to the latter's undisguised joy. Occasionally it was a large bird of some kind on free flight round the room which was returned to a large cage upon my arrival.

"Let him free!" I would cry.

"Oh, he doesn't like men," was the response.

"Never mind, let's see what happens."

By this time the main objective had been achieved anyway. On one such visit, I already felt an intimate member of the household, but it was too late and the bird was released. It was of the cockatoo family and it flew a couple of circuits round the room, making low passes at my head. It was clearly making up its mind as to my sex and therefore preparing to be spurned or befriended. Unfortunately, its ability to determine sex in my case was faulty, and it suddenly alighted on my balding head, slithering about as it attempted to obtain a grip (painful to me). As it slithered around, the strain was too much for its cloaca, and I was aware of some 'foreign' matter on my head. What could one do? To strike out would have alienated my developing friendship with the household, so I attempted to make life as uncomfortable for the bird as it was for me by alternatively tipping my head, first to one side, then to the other, in the hope of persuading the bird that there were better places for roosting. This was all to no avail, for it slithered about, occasionally flapping its wings and at one point even gripped my right ear in an attempt to obtain a foothold. I only escaped by excusing myself to go to the bathroom which I hoped would be 'off-limits' (it was), where I had a mini-shower. When I returned, the bird was sulking in a corner of its cage: it never spoke except to squawk 'Foxtrot Oscar' as I was leaving. I paused, and caught a glint in my patient's eyes, whilst his wife looked pleased.

"Isn't he clever?" she said.

Her husband (who was an amputee) whispered to me, "Of course she doesn't understand what the old bird is saying nor for that matter, does he. I used to be in the police; you will understand," giving me a knowing wink!

The privilege of being admitted not just into a household, but as an intimate, if temporary member of a household is probably restricted to ministers of religion and my own profession. Social workers, home helps and others may see families intimately, but on a somewhat more restricted basis related to their duties. It is a privilege which enables one to appreciate how the real world lives, or, more often, how the disadvantaged world exists. It is a world which politicians in their pomposity do not know exists, and so, in their distanced ways, they are quite unable to comprehend the feelings of a sizeable portion of the electorate. It is a world where real feelings are felt when real problems have to be tackled, problems such as warmth, food, and hygiene, and where the meaning of self-reliance is evident, or the consequences suffered.

One patient put it succinctly. "These politicians are an ignorant, arrogant lot, they fob us off with a lot of statistics, which they assume we will lap up. Where they are so stupid is that they pass statistics off as information when what we need is knowledge or an understanding of that information. Even a halfwit can perceive that our own knowledge about our lives bears little resemblance to the official statistics meted out."

I can say with conviction that I made 10,000 friends during those years, and they represent one of the most satisfying tasks in my whole life. A few examples might be of interest.

Take One – Lights, Music:

In this instance the patient was a 15-year-old girl with a psychotic background, living with her father in a deprived part of the city of Gloucester. The examination called for a semi-intimate examination of the girl's thighs (she suffered from uncorrected Perthe's disease of her left hip). The two of them lived in a neglected two-roomed 'apartment', sparsely furnished but with a varied assortment of video equipment of every kind, including three video cameras mounted on their tripods, and high-intensity lighting, as then unlit. I sensed a potentially dangerous situation, which was confirmed when the father announced that he intended to record the whole interview, including the physical examination. I countered with some excuse and had to escape as quickly as I could when the father threatened to call the police. I felt the boot was on the wrong foot, for I still believe that the equipment was obtained criminally. As I left I learned as an unsuspecting innocent party how easy it is to be made to feel the guilty party by a professional criminal, or, for that matter, a professional interrogator as well.

It illustrated, to me at least, how important the 'right to silence' is to those who might find themselves in police custody.

The Silent Guilt

Tom and Jane, both in their late twenties, had managed to buy their dream home in the rural countryside of Gloucestershire, between Cheltenham and Cirencester. They had conducted their lives with care, waiting to rear a family until they reckoned they could afford it. Their first child was a boy, christened James, who appeared to be in perfect health. Some two years later their second child, Alan, was also born, also apparently healthy. However, whilst Jane was carrying this second child they noticed that James' gait did not seem quite as it should be and that he appeared to lack energy. They sought advice and were referred to a paediatrician who was horrified to discover after tests that the youngster was suffering from an unusual form of muscular dystrophy which was affecting the use of his muscles. Much worse, and the parents had to be told, he would be unlikely to reach maturity before dying from this illness, probably before he reached the age of ten.

Worse was to come: whilst Tom was quite healthy and to all outward intents, so was Jane, she was the carrier of the deadly gene which was the cause of the trouble, and already another child was on the way. Would it be a boy? If a girl then the chances were that she would be all right, though possibly also a carrier of the gene. In these circumstances though, at least a stop might be put to passing the problem further by suitable sterilisation.

As fate decided, the second child was also a boy. By the time I saw the family the first child was virtually immobilised, though old enough to understand what was the matter with him, and the second boy had not yet learned to walk but was progressing. Thus three of the four members of that family knew what lay in store, and collectively they were preparing themselves for what lay ahead. In due course the two parents would be left alone, and, more significantly, the cause of the problem, Jane, knew she was inadvertently responsible.

I often thought about this family, and one day, some 5 years later, I was driving along the road from Cirencester to Cheltenham, when I noticed a 'For Sale' notice outside that same house. I feared the worst – it would be about now when the second boy would be nearing the end of his life. I did not think it was my business to enquire directly.

Some three years later I chanced on Jane and Tom shopping in Cirencester and noticed that they were pushing a pram and another boy was walking alongside. They remembered me and stopped to explain that they had not felt able to go on living at their old home after both their boys had died, but had now adopted two boys and here was the result!

I felt that out of tragedy had been effected some form of rescue for two good people; I felt elated and that a load had been lifted.

For Queen And Country:

I saw this case in London, East Sussex Gardens to be exact, not far from Marble Arch. It was in a modern-looking block of flats which had been taken over by the Westminster Housing Department to house some of the people on their books. Whenever a telephone number was given in the application documents, I phoned to make an appointment. All I knew was that the applicant, a man in his late 50s, said he was unable to walk without assistance, 'due to leg trouble'. He was gruff and sounded resentful when I spoke to him on the phone, but he had an educated voice.

I arranged to call on him that evening, after finishing my day at the St John Ambulance HQ (I was the chief commander at this time). I had little difficulty in locating the block of flats, and noted that at least there was a lift in the building. As instructed I let myself into his apartment, noticing as I did so a pungent smell of pipe tobacco. As I entered his sitting room he greeted me with a resentful look, and I suspected that he was embarrassed at his privacy being invaded. He was sitting in a chair with one leg resting on a foot stool; the other leg was not visible. The room was sparsely furnished with a bed in the corner and a wheelchair by the chair in which he sat. As I shook his hand I noticed that he was 'on the square', with certain documentation by his side confirming the fact.

It turned out that he had lived there for a about a year, had recently had his left leg amputated above the knee and now felt unable to get used to his prosthesis, which was standing in a corner. He was clearly a bad-tempered man (but then, wouldn't I be too in his predicament) and I tried to be as patient as possible as he told his story. (His wife had left him some months previously, but I felt that was none of my business and so didn't ask questions on that score.)

The examination being nearly complete, I asked him for certain documentary evidence and he reached to a nearby table and picked up a small wooden box. As he opened it I noticed the ribbon of the Military Cross and also a red ribbon with the vertical thin white stripes of the Order of the British Empire, so I asked him about them. Perhaps because he realised that I recognised their significance he opened up. Serving during World War II in North Africa (where he won the MC) and finishing as a captain, he had taken an extended commission, ending in Washington on the staff of the British Joint Services Mission. There he had been awarded the MBE for his liaison with the Pentagon over arms shipments.

As he grew older, he said, he had probably begun drinking too much, and this, together with his heavy smoking (his wife was an asthmatic), led to his marital breakdown. Then he lost his leg through the arteries 'furring up' and 'here I am'.

His story was not uncommon. It is an example of how some of our heroes had not been able to move with the times and had developed slight chips on their shoulders, and things go from bad to worse.

On leaving I was able to get in touch with an army benevolent society and they put him into a suitable home. I read of his death some time later, but I like to think that more came of my visit than simply getting him a few extra pounds a week on account of his disability.

The Light That Flickered

Whilst serving in the rank of Surgeon Commander, in the Royal Navy, I was appointed to Farnborough to conduct airborne medical experiments, which provided opportunities to fly many different types of (by the standards then prevailing) high-performance aircraft.

Amongst many other interesting subjects, I became involved in human causes of aircraft accidents – human error is still the commonest cause, even today, of aviation mishaps.

One particular fatality has remained vividly in my mind to this day, not so much for what caused the accident, so much as what emerged during the consequent researches into the cause. It is appropriate to report this case here.

It was during the summer of 1953 when I was asked to investigate the circumstances of a fatal helicopter crash which had just happened at the Royal Navy Air Station at Gosport, in Hampshire. The pilot was well-known to me as a competent, indeed experienced fixed wing pilot, and had been halfway through a course which would qualify him to fly helicopters.

I arranged to visit the scene of the fatal crash, and asked to fly a machine of the same type and re-enact the same exercise as the deceased pilot had been carrying out. He had been flying solo, and conducting a simulated engine failure, involving climbing to about 1000 feet, before closing the engine throttle, and so simulating a failed engine.

Without going into the technicalities, this would involve turning into the wind before closing the throttle and, like a sycamore leaf failing from a tree, the helicopter would descend at a steady rate, being sustained by the rotating rotors. At a given height from the ground, to cushion his landing, the pilot would normally alter the 'pitch' of the rotor blades with a slight hand movement on the throttle grip. For some reason, he had failed to carry out this simple action, and had plummeted into the ground and been killed.

A perusal of the meteorological conditions prevailing on the day of the accident revealed that on the fateful day it had been hot, with a light breeze from the south, which meant that the exercise would have been conducted heading in that direction, and with no cloud cover, and, being midday, the hot sun would have been directly overhead at the time of the accident.

Coincidentally, conditions were similar on the day when I simulated the flight – no cloud, warm, and a light southerly breeze taking the worst of the heat from the overhead midday sun. The rotor blades rotated immediately above the pilot's head, and could be seen rotating through the clear perspex canopy top. I noted this, and took off to commence the simulation. At 1000 feet, I turned into wind – and, heading south, closed the throttle to simulate engine failure.

As the rotor blades slowed with the loss of power, I got an overwhelming sense of *déjà vu*, distracting my attention from the task in hand: my attention wandered, not helped by a virtual kaleidoscope of colours dancing in front of my eyes. I was recalling flying a Spitfire, landing on the main runway at Farnborough, towards the west, into an already low setting sun. As I had closed the throttle, and was gently lifting the nose to settle into a three-point landing, the sun was obscuring forward vision with a myriad of colour as the rays of the sun were broken up by the now idling five-bladed propeller of the Spitfire's Griffon engine. I had had difficulty in concentrating on the task of maintaining the aircraft's landing run on a straight course. I felt pleasantly relaxed, almost disembodied, when suddenly my attention was brought back to the immediate need to alter the helicopter's remorseless descent towards the ground, and I gave a sharp twist to the rotor lever, and the aircraft settled onto the ground – reasonably gently, but leaving me perspiring rather too freely.

The mystery of my colleague's death had been explained, but there was a need to discover more about what turned out to be 'the flicker effect', which many people will recognise having experienced themselves, for example when watching telegraph poles 'flick' at a specified interval as when viewed from a train, or when exposed to a stroboscopic light at a dance, or whilst watching a television picture.

My further researches took me to meet Dr Graham Walter, who was working at the time at the Burden Institute, near Bristol. He was not surprised at my story, as he estimated that some 3% of the population are susceptible to the effects of 'flicker', when a source of light was being interrupted at specific rate, so as to 'clash' with the brain impulses. He likened it to neurological resonance, and, in extreme cases, it could precipitate an epileptiform attack.

What was even more fascinating, however, was to learn of some further research which Dr Walter was then conducting into the analysis and categorisation of the alpha rhythms of the brain, which, he believed, could be categorised into specific types, in much the same way as blood groups are segregated. He believed that by such analysis, it would be possible to forecast potential, and so far inexplicable 'personality clashes', with their attendant problems, and only to put 'brain rhythm compatible' personalities in close working proximity to one another.

It might also explain why an individual who has two close friends, and wishes to make up a happy, compatible trio is astonished to find when, on introducing them, that they 'spark' together– much as incompatible blood groups are disastrous if transfused.

Sadly, Dr Walters died shortly afterwards, before – so far as I am aware – completing his researches, though I did note that he and his, to my mind, excellent assistant appeared unable to hold a civil discussion together!

How Dare You!

The questions on the form for attendance allowance were far-reaching and detailed. They were calculated to ascertain how much assistance the applicant required in connection, to a large extent, with carrying out bodily functions such as undressing, getting into bed, bathing, and even feeding. Some cases would need supervision to avoid danger to themselves, even though they did not require assistance with their routine bodily habits. One such case was that of Janette, who lived in a terraced house in Swindon.

I saw from her application form that she was an unstable diabetic, and having made an appointment, rang her front doorbell one spring morning. I was not prepared, however, for the unusual beauty of a 30-year-old woman who came to the door with well-groomed hair, dressed in a smart frock. I noticed two things, however, which detracted from what I saw.

First, her eyes were not looking at mine, but, with a sort of far away detached look, they were looking over my right shoulder. The second thing which I noticed was that the colours of her skirt clashed with the colours of a scarf tied round her neck, as though she had not chosen very carefully.

That was it, I thought to myself, she was blind and diabetic? Yes, I remembered her application form and what it had said. Diagnosis? Easy: diabetic retinopathy!

As I spoke to her her eyes came near to meeting mine, though still with a detached look in spite of the welcoming smile. I followed her in to her sitting room where she beckoned me to sit on the sofa, before sitting alongside me, but not before a Yorkshire terrier had jumped up, placing itself between us and looking anxiously first at his mistress then suspiciously at me, growling slightly at the same time. 'A good minder,' I mused.

Janette and I quickly completed the questionnaire. It was clear that Janette was quite unable to monitor her own urine for sugar, nor subsequently to measure out the requisite amount of insulin twice a day to combat the blood sugar, the result of her diabetes. Had she ever been admitted to hospital as an emergency? Yes, on several occasions, and thus was the case made out for her needing 'attention to prevent danger to herself'. 'Straightforward,' I thought as I prepared to sign the medical examination report. But I had not finished, for there were several, now superfluous questions which had to be completed.

"That's nearly all," I said. "Would you be able to go upstairs, get undressed and get into bed..." My voice trailed away in embarrassment, "No, perhaps we should take each question one at a time!"

As a postscript, Janette's case was turned down, why I don't know, but it was only one of two cases for which I was asked to do a second visit; at my suggestion she had lodged an appeal. I was pleased to hear that on this second occasion it was accepted that Janette met the criteria for requiring 'attention to prevent herself getting into danger'.

'Bottoms Up'

It was consoling to find that very few of the patients I visited were 'trying to get something for nothing'. The extremely small number who clearly did not meet the strict conditions laid down to qualify for attendance allowance had applied in ignorance, many having been encouraged by social workers or friends.

It was also rewarding to find that one was remembered many years later for having visited an area. So it was in Swindon, in a district I knew well from earlier visits, when I called at a certain house. As I knocked on the door a neighbour came out of her own house and called me by name, to my surprise.

"How nice to see you again, Doctor; I'm afraid Mrs Jones [whom I had come to see] has been sent to hospital."

I thanked her and she continued, "Of course, you remember visiting Mother two years ago." I had to confess that I was not quite sure that I did, but tactfully enquired as to how she was.

"I'm afraid Mother passed away some time ago but she always talked about you; she always said she had never had her bottom wiped by a young man before."

It appeared that this old girl had been in heart failure when I called, and was unable to take herself to the loo. I must have seen that she was uncomfortable, and had apparently helped her along to the loo, turned her round, before hoisting her knickers clear and placing her adequate bottom over the hole; then leaving her till she was ready before cleaning her up and getting her back to her chair.

Such an incident may be all in a day's work, but it is gratifying to learn that such a small gesture can leave a pleasant, lasting impression.

Arrest That Man:

Not all the cases I called on were unreservedly welcoming. One case on the outskirts of Birmingham refused to allow me into his flat until he had called the police, and he was extremely hostile until they arrived, in spite of my reassurances and providing means of identifying myself.

Apparently he had been burgled twice, and assaulted once by an impostor posing as a doctor. He was clearly in a very suspicious frame of mind, but I felt a deal of pity for him and wondered whether the police are always directed to the right targets in need of protection.

'Fings Ain't Always What They Seem.'

There is an area some two miles from Paddington station, north of the Harrow Road in London, not far from where the Notting Hill Carnival is held, which might be a thousand miles from London, such is the Caribbean atmosphere created. It is a district which would seem to have its own laws, and there 'foreigners' are regarded with suspicion. It is an underworld of its own and a stranger goes there at his peril, especially after dark.

Many of my cases lived within its boundaries and I always paid my visits on foot. I also wore what I felt were inconspicuous, as well as being rather shabby clothes. In the shadows I could see vague figures, and once was knocked brusquely to one side by a man wearing a stocking mask hurrying about whatever his business might be. It might have been the setting for Dr Jekyll and Mr Hyde, and yet if I had to ask for directions I was always treated with a form of courtesy, if suspicion. I learned to avoid eye contact as this suggested aggression.

I had arranged to call on one particular case at about 7.30 p.m. one autumn evening, when, just to add to the drama, there was a thick choking fog making it difficult to find one's way through the streets. It was noticeable that there was a high percentage of abandoned cars clogging the already narrow roadways. The address I was seeking was difficult to locate, and as I paced back and forth I felt that I was re-enacting a scene more appropriate to the Victorian days of Jack the Ripper or Sherlock Holmes. Absorbed in such thoughts, I was surprised when I was addressed by a policeman who was dressed in the modern way; I half expected him to blow a whistle, in keeping with my imagination.

"Can I help you?" He then added, almost as an afterthought, "Sir." (maybe he had assessed me as a 'visitor'.)

I showed him my papers with the address of my patient.

"Oh, yes, she doesn't get many visitors. Is she expecting you? She lives down those steps, in the basement. I usually call on her once a week just to make sure that she's all right." As I reflected on this scene I felt a reassurance that with all the talk today about police not knowing their 'clientele', this was refreshing.

I went down the steps to my patient; the door was unlocked, and I entered, to be met in the narrow hallway by my patient, a women of about 75, in a wheelchair.

"Follow me," she said in an educated voice. I noticed that she was wearing freshly applied lipstick and a little rouge. 'A proud woman,' I thought. 'And clearly anticipating my call.'

I followed her into the only room, so far as I discovered, which was dimly lit and looked as though it had been excavated from the floor of Vesuvius, for it was covered uniformly in a mantle of grey dust. I say uniformly, but to be exact, tracks had been made in the dust to mark 'runs' from a double bed with grey sheets on it, to the door, and to a fireplace which housed a gas fire. A broken-down chair and an ancient standard lamp plus a commode and a large bookcase filled with books were the only other items of furniture in the room. What took my attention though, was that although there were the remains of what looked like an Axminster carpet, worn threadbare with the repeated rolling of the wheelchair, there was no room for anything else in the way of furniture. The remainder of the floor was occupied by bundles of *The Times*, neatly bundled into stacks about 10 inches high. I glanced at the dates and saw some faded editions going back to the late 60s. Clearly this was an interesting character.

After completing my report (she had a double amputation, one above, and the other just below the knee), I listened to her story, which she clearly wanted to recount, for she had few visitors apart from her home help, who came twice a week and also did her shopping. She hadn't been out of her flat for about ten years, except for her monthly visits to nearby St Mary's Hospital. She had turned into a recluse and her only direct contact with the outside world was by way of a radio and, she wanted to explain, "my friend the local bobby, John, who looks in occasionally. I used to love my books, and was an avid writer to *The Times*, but I'm ready to go now."

She fell silent, as though inviting me to encourage her to talk. Then, "I see your name is 'Ellis'. Don't suppose you are any relation to a colleague of mine in the FANYs? Her name was Baxter Ellis."

I could hardly believe it, for Mary Baxter Ellis (she was known as 'Dick') was my great aunt and we had been very close; she had been a very senior officer in the FANYs. I was able to tell this new-found friend of mine something about what had happened since the war. In fact this old lady had been operating in occupied France with people like Odette, so I recounted some confirmation that the FANYs were indeed known to the Germans, and had caused them certain inconveniences. My aunt had attended the Nuremberg War Crime Trials with Sir Hartley Shawcross. She was wearing her uniform with 'FANY' as a 'flash' on her shoulder. During a break in the trial she happened to be close to Hermann Goering who, on seeing the word 'FANY', stopped in his tracks and, as his face became distorted with rage, he hissed, "FANY!" before moving on!

As I recounted the story of how Goering had clearly found the activities of certain branches of the FANYs 'troublesome', I could see that my reclusive patient was emerging from her self-imposed isolation from the outside world. Her eyes were brightening as she revelled in some of the memories which my tale had stirred.

I gently encouraged her to talk, and the story of her life in many ways epitomised what so many of her generation had gone through and yet in a way created. I reflected as she talked that she, and so many of her contemporaries, had made a contribution to the very way of life which we today benefit from and are able to enjoy if we so choose.

It transpired that, soon after the war finished, she had married an ex-RAF pilot, who, like so many of his comrades, had found it difficult to adjust to the quieter ways of peace. Restless, he had failed in some respects to face the realities of a post-war world and strived to continue with his flying in various ways, yet at the same time failed to find satisfaction, resulting in his personality becoming increasingly difficult to live with. Thus there were two casualties from the war, not just himself, but also my patient who was recounting her own story and subsequent mishaps.

After certain happenings which I did not pursue, he became a test pilot, emigrating to Los Angeles and flying for the Douglas Aircraft Corporation. At about this time, it must have been in the late 60s, my patient could stand it no more and left him, returning to London, at first endeavouring to write but then turning into a recluse in the state in which I found her.

There were no children so my patient was left to fall back on her own meagre resources and she somehow fell between all the Social Services grants because she had lived abroad for a number of critical years.

She is an example, and there are many, of how a combination of age and chance can cause an elderly person to be left behind, stranded like flotsam left on the high waterline as the tide of life continues to ebb and flow. Some persons drift into such receptacles as 'homes for the elderly', others get left behind like stranded whales until they die, welcoming any attention that might come their way.

As I left her I pondered as to how much she had contributed to their joint downfall, for no one party can be held wholly responsible for a marital breakdown. Alas I shall never know.

Incommunicado

When astronauts are returning to earth they go through a period, during the critical stage of re-entering the earth's atmosphere, when communication between the spacecraft and control at base ceases. The men at control find this a most tense period.

In the sick room a similar situation can arise, as, for example, in people who have suffered a stroke who may have lost their ability to speak. They know what they want to say, but the 'exclusive' part of the speech centre has gone dead. Frequently, the victim, due to frustration, will become irritable and often enraged, thus acquiring the reputation of being 'difficult', unless a great deal of patience and understanding is practised. Under current pressure for productivity in most branches of work the last place to demand this is in the sick room, and when dealing with such patients. Haste when nursing and caring for ill people would be totally counter-productive.

The worst possible scenario, which I have frequently witnessed, is when the carer treats the patient like an idiot, the worst version of 'Does he take sugar' syndrome, treating the stroke victim as though he is an imbecile, which he certainly is not. All he needs is to be treated with dignity and patience. He may be slow, but, given time, he will find ways of conveying his thoughts and needs. Establish a way of communicating ('Nod your head if you want to say 'yes'' is a type of primitive communication), and the patient will respond as though he has been let in from a foreign planet.

What A Bloody Mess.

Before I called I already knew that the patient I was to see in a flat near West Bromwich was on routine dialysis due to kidney failure. What I did not know was that the patient had just recently been discharged from hospital to continue his dialysis at home with the help of his wife. Such cases are an example of the marvels of modern medicine, and, with suitable training, enables people with total kidney failure, who would have died under conditions of not many years ago, to lead a virtually normal life, providing that they spend six hours three times a week connected up to a sophisticated artificial kidney machine. This procedure calls for considerable skills on the part of the carer (usually a spouse, or parent in the case of a child), who must supervise the circulation of the blood repeatedly through the machine and take blood pressure readings etc., at regular intervals. Continuity of attention during the transfusion is essential and this calls for special electricity supplies in case of power failures. Though no surgery is called for during the dialysis procedure it calls for a high level of technical knowledge, and things *can* go wrong, as this case was to demonstrate.

I rang the doorbell of the flat. A female voice, with some tone of distress I noted, shouted, asking me to wait a minute as she was 'rather busy'.

After about four minutes, I found that the door was open and entered. On going upstairs I was horrified at what I found.

The room contained a black couple; he was connected to a dialysis machine and his wife, dressed in a theatre gown with surgical gloves was striving to reconnect the cannula in the man's arm. There was a considerable amount of blood about, so I stripped off my coat, rolled up my sleeves, found the bathroom and quickly scrubbed up as though for an operation. No time for gloves (there weren't any) so I broke surgical rule No. 1 regarding AIDS and tackled the situation, with the wife assisting. Nothing very technical was necessary; all that was required was to apply a tourniquet, re-connect the cannula, release the tourniquet and check the blood pressure (I suspect it was kept up by the excitement, as the patient was taking a keen interest in what was going on; after all, he had a vested interest!). We enjoyed a refreshing cup of tea as the dialysis was resumed and I made out my report. The competence of that young couple earned my respect and admiration; I hadn't really noticed they were black, except that his veins were slightly more difficult to find, and I pondered, not for the first time, how and why racism could exist in our society. I certainly was never aware of any racial distinction or animosity amongst the medical cases I visited, of whatever colour or creed. As I left I felt a glow of satisfaction in that I had been able to make a minor contribution that day, and felt that medicine could, on occasions, make some days very worthwhile.

One Hell of a Mess!

The notes told me that the man I was going to visit in a market town in Dorset was 43, and had been operated on recently for cancer of his bowel. The information was, as usual, fairly scant, and I reflected on how one needed to watch for any further clues which could lead to a more accurate diagnosis, for it was not unusual for patients to be entirely ignorant as to their illness. If I was to visit somebody I made a point of trying to phone first, not only to make an appointment but to establish contact. Even without mentioning illness it was surprising how often something would be said which lead one to make a diagnosis. A good example was multiple sclerosis, which, amongst other things, can lead to a slight slurring of speech, discernible even before it has been noticed by the family.

I arrived at a block of flats where my next patient with bowel trouble lived on the 3rd floor. Through the security speaker at the front door I was instructed to come to come up in the lift, but thought I could perceive a note of anxiety in the man's voice. It transpired that he lived alone and, on entering his living room I found him sitting on a sofa with no clothes on below his waist and in a terrible mess.

He apologised, explaining that he had only recently had his colostomy (the bowel is brought through the skin just below the navel) and he had not yet known how to look after it properly. As a result of some fizzy beer the night before (to celebrate his homecoming) his bowels had become somewhat active, bursting through his colostomy bag and running all over his clothes and the sofa, where he sat contemplating what to do next.

I stripped off my coat, rolled up my sleeves, took my tie off (with hindsight, I am not sure why I did this, but vaguely thought it might get 'involved'), got a bowl of warm water a large towel, and started to clean things up, at the same time stemming the flow.

I became aware that the room was getting darker and at the same time there was a scraping sound from outside the window opposite the sofa where my patient and I were getting on with our task.

Then to my horror I saw the top side of a ladder being pushed up to the window and realised that soon that this would be followed by a hand and a face.

"Oh dear," said my patient, "I'd forgotten its the day for the window cleaner and I will have to pay him." My mind was on a much more serious matter than how to pay the window cleaner. When he got to our window, how would he react to the sight which greeted him? Would he faint and fall off his ladder? If so, what damage would he sustain? Would I be to blame, was my subscription to the Medical Defence Union paid up? Might I even be stuck off the Medical Register for lack of care?

I seized the towel and held it up in front of us, so that the window cleaner, on reaching window level, gazed in with an astonished expression on his face as he surveyed the scene. What he must have seen would be a couple of semi-naked men sitting together on a sofa, caught in an act (could it be properly described 'of indecency'? 'Consenting adults' in private?). As I watched him for a moment, he transfixed with a dripping sponge in one hand, his bucket fell to the ground some thirty feet below with a loud clatter. I heard a voice below yelling,

"Must you be so careless? That just missed me!" This brought him back to reality and he disappeared down the ladder, followed shortly afterwards by the ladder being removed.

I never saw him again, but resumed my primary task, and soon the patient and I were finished, properly dressed and enjoying a well-earned cuppa. I felt that another patient was not wholly displeased with the overall outcome of the visit.

Fit?

Although in the pursuit of one's medical career there are to be found light-hearted, even hilarious moments, epilepsy can only very rarely be regarded in this vein. Epilepsy is but one, though an important one, of a group of diseases which are far-reaching in the disproportional effect which they exert on the social, professional and working life of an otherwise perfectly normal, healthy person.

Epilepsy is one of earliest identifiable medical conditions, and reference to it can be found in the New Testament. Chapter IX, describing an epileptic boy as being in the grip of the devil, tells how he gives a sharp cry and foams at the mouth, and describes the prehistoric practice of trephining the skull to cut out the demon which has taken possession of the individual.

The more one studies epilepsy, the more difficult it becomes to understand it. An impression is gained that one is peering into the human equivalent of extra-terrestrial exploration and attempting to pry into the very soul of man, perhaps even linking up with the largely forgotten (by *Homo sapiens*) realm of extrasensory perception.

Types of epilepsy range right across the neurological spectrum. There is the classic *grand mal* epileptic fit, sometimes preceded by a warning and sometimes not, when, like a massive thunderstorm, all the available forces are unleased in the neurological universe. Such a massive release of electrical discharge within the brain might well be described as a neurological orgasm, and lasts but a brief time, being measured in seconds rather than minutes. Like a thunderstorm, it is not in itself usually harmful, but the results can be devastating, even, albeit rarely, fatal, as in the case of one of my patients who suffocated on his pillow during a nocturnal attack.

The massive electrical discharge in the brain during the fit puts every muscle in the body into spasm. It is this which causes the typical epileptic cry which causes such distress to a witness, but none to the victim, for he is unconscious and his thought processes in limbo. The cry is caused by the respiratory muscles contracting, pulling in air through the already contracting vocal chords. Similarly, the bladder may empty, with embarrassing social consequences.

Like the thunderstorm, this period quickly passes as the body's increasing need for oxygen reasserts itself. After a brief period when the arms and legs thrash purposelessly, the fit passes, leaving the victim physically exhausted but peaceful, with no worse symptoms than possibly a slight headache and a desire to sleep, and no awareness of the dramatic events which have just taken place.

So much for the classic *grand mal* attack. There are as many variants and lesser versions of epileptic attacks as there are of thunderstorms, right down to the cerebral equivalent of the northern lights, the *petit mal* epileptic attack lasting perhaps one or two seconds, which is totally and irretrievably removed from the victim's memory; this experience can be likened to watching a film from which a dozen or so frames have been removed, leaving the viewer (or victim) to pick up the thread as best he can. Other variants may not interrupt consciousness or awareness, but a limb or other part of the body may twitch or jerk, indicating localised electrical activity in the part of the brain controlling that part of the body (Jacksonian epilepsy).

There are strict guidelines laid down for anybody with a history of epilepsy, but we need not concern ourselves with these at this point.

There are also bizarre forms of the affliction, for example, attacks may take the form of uncontrollable laughter, or a compulsion to fall asleep (narcolepsy).

Of greater import is a form which may not be apparent to any watching person, and, unless appropriate tests are carried out, may never be diagnosed. This is a state of automatism, which may last for a considerable period of time, during which the victim may carry out deeds totally foreign to his nature, and not be aware of his actions. These may or may not follow any visible evidence of anything untoward.

It was with these thoughts in mind that I called at a house in Swindon to see a man in his early twenties with a known history of epilepsy. The local police knew him, following an episode when he had apparently gone berserk in a china shop, causing extensive damage.

I met him, an apparently normal, pleasant young man with an apologetic manner, and clearly part of a close family with his mother and three siblings, the youngest of whom was about 12. It was clear that they were all very conversant with their epileptic brother, and were keen to be present during any questioning, for they were quite open about the matter, including the 'breaking-up' of the china shop, of which the victim had no recollection, the cause having been accepted as post-epileptic automatism.

My task, however, was to record all the facts for another purpose: to ascertain his entitlement to an attendance allowance, so I took a normal full history, asking relevant questions, of which one was to establish whether there was any warning of an impending attack. The victim said he never got any warning, so I asked his mother, as mothers often recognise signs in their children which nobody else does, a form of maternal 'cloning'.

No; neither the mother nor any member of the family had ever noticed any warning signs prior to an attack, which would start with anything ranging from minor shaking of a limb right through to falling to the ground and then following the typical course of an epileptic attack. This stage would be followed usually by normal recovery, but, on occasions, the victim would be unaware of his actions and go into a dazed state, a form of automatism, undergoing a personality change and doing things completely at variance with his normal character. It was during this phase that he was liable to run amok, and, on occasions, involve the police, as when he broke up the china shop.

Having ascertained that no member of the family got any warning of a pending attack, the 12-year-old girl suddenly said,

"But she knows," pointing to a large Alsatian bitch which was stretched in front of the fire near her master.

Fascinated, I pressed the little girl for more details,

"When John [her brother] is going to have a turn, Lassie [it seemed an appropriate name for the dog in view of what followed] knows that something is wrong, she will prick up her ears, raise her head, as though 'listening' for something, then will get up and, standing on her hind legs, will put her front paws on John's shoulders, as though trying to make him sit down."

The rest of my visit is history, but I reflected, on driving home, that here was yet another example of 'something' which we humans have largely lost through disuse, a form of extrasensory perception (ESP).

On looking back over these cases, I realise that I got more satisfaction from this phase of my medical career than any other, probably because illness and death can be great forces for bringing individuals to a common level. No longer is there any place for pomp or posturing, only scope for dignity. Debilitating illness and the final days of life are great levellers, and it has been a privilege to have known so many when the final 'count' takes place. I can imagine no better way to feel the pulse of the community.

The elderly are, generally speaking, a happy breed. They no longer fear death, but only the way in which they might die – in pain, with a loss of dignity or in need of assistance towards the end. All the more reason why one should ensure that one makes a 'Living Will' (See Chapter Eighteen) so that one's wishes are known and can be carried out when the time comes. Paradoxically, the only time in life when death is feared is when it is least likely to occur, when one is young.

I have left what is probably the most significant illness, in that it is a threat to the whole human race, to the last in recounting examples of cases. I refer to ACQUIRED IMMUNE DEFICIENCY SYNDROME (AIDS) (see Chapter Thirteen).

Anyone For AIDS?

I deliberately pose this question: there is no way by which you can identify whether someone is HIV positive by simply meeting them. You may well suspect that they could be by their appearance (but not always), or their lifestyle, or just have a 'hunch', but this is not evidence, simply 'think-say'. The only way to diagnose AIDS is to *think* AIDS and then to conduct an examination along these lines.

Even when a colleague on a committee of which I was a member became so ill he had to be sent home because of a very heavy 'flu-like' cold, even when he could hardly walk, I was fooled, and it was not until I heard that he was on a life-support machine that I realised what I had missed, and I was at that time seeing three or four cases a month of fully developed AIDS-related illnesses.

So when I received the application papers to visit a case in the Bayswater Road I was put on my guard for two reasons: first, the district seemed to be a reception area for terminal AIDS-related illnesses (I had seen over 40 cases in the Paddington and Bayswater districts) and second, the applicant was a 28-year-old male who said, when I telephoned him, that he would be unable to get out of bed to let me in when I called.

I arrived by arrangement very early in the morning. The address turned out to be a semi-basement flat in quite an elegant street. The door was open, so I entered and was summoned by my patient calling me into a pleasant bedroom. It was a tidy, clean room with a double bed on which my patient was lying, a dressing table and two chairs, and it was nicely decorated (with little feminine touches), making for a homely atmosphere.

My patient turned out to be a fresh, pale-complexioned young man who was markedly thin and clearly in some distress, caused by his bowels being loose; this can be a characteristic of the illness. I noticed that his toenails had candida (significantly) and he also had an unproductive cough as though he had a cold.

He was forthcoming and revealed that he had known he was HIV positive for some years, but it was only in the last few months that he had become very weak and now needed help to get to the lavatory (I had noticed a commode by his bed).

I proceeded with the examination, which was brief, as the situation was clear. As with so many other cases, I felt a certain satisfaction in that I felt no inclination to condemn; he was to me a patient, a human being, and my desire was simply to be sympathetic to his plight and to do whatever I was able to help him in his final days (he died some eight weeks later).

The surprise came towards the end of my examination. The bedroom door opened, and a man in his late thirties came in, bade me good morning and then proceeded to the dressing table, gathering a few oddments, including some loose change which he put into his pocket, much as any man might do after dressing and before setting out for the office. I then noticed that he was dressed in a black jacket with striped trousers with a white shirt and collar and a grey tie. I was so taken aback that I said, "You look as though you are going to appear in court."

"You are correct; I am defending a minor criminal this morning," he replied, and disappeared out into the street.

My patient, with a look of pride mixed with sadness, explained that his lover was a partner in a well-known firm of solicitors in the City.

I shall never forget this case, with its poignant overtones reminding one that truth is stranger than fiction. If we stopped to think before passing judgement the world might be an easier place to understand, for it seems that today compassion is all too frequently at a premium.

Conclusion

Perhaps the saddest aspect of AIDS is not that it invariably has a fatal, if deferred ending, but that during this extended period of illness the victim is so often ostracised by his family just at the very time when family support is vital. It is the one time in life that forgiveness is essential, and yet I saw so many terminal cases, not to mention those still in a 'healthy' way of life, who had crept to the oblivion and anonymous refuge of London where they could hide their shame and loneliness.

At no time did I feel anything but compassion for these cases, and derived considerable satisfaction from the fact that, to me, they were patients in need of help, and, just as rewarding, that they appreciated being treated as human beings.

Domestic Roulette: Till Death Us Do Part (For better or for Worse).

There are several justifiable reasons for including a specimen case history of divorce.

Firstly, it is one of the more common causes of stress, scoring 73 points on the 'stress table', and the second highest of those causes listed.

Secondly, the resulting distress is not self-confining, affecting whole families even unto second and third generations, and to this degree is self-perpetuating.

Thirdly, it is a sad reflection on modern society's 'civilisation' achievement, now affecting nearly one in two marriages. To this end, Richard Curtis got the ratio about right when he wrote *Four Weddings and a Funeral.*

Lastly, the oblique reference to death in the marital wedding vows would appear to offer a further opportunity to 'cheat' death by the relatively simple expedient of untying the knot, though this course would seem to create more problems as well as sadness (akin to grief), than it solves.

So, for better or for worse, the problem is now addressed by recounting the case history of such a victim who was a patient of mine. The story is as told by my patient to me in his own words. I have called it *Domestic Roulette.*

Though not strictly medical, it has certain medical overtones, and illustrates how a marital separation or divorce may well precipitate a medical condition, such as shingles, for example. Medical conditions can also underlie a divorce, or, surprisingly, can also bring previously divorced couples together again, by releasing the very tension between couples of strong incompatible personalities.

This then is the case of the destruction of a marriage as recalled by a husband.

I will call my couple Arthur and Sheila. They had both been married previously. They were both professional people, in fact Sheila was a barrister, and thus had knowledge of the law.

They were both victims of the stresses and demands made on individuals by modern society, which accounted for the breakdown of their first marriages. In the case of Arthur stress arose from the need to produce a financial harvest in excess of that which his professional skills were able to meet; in the case of Sheila, stress came from a conflict between her ambition to pursue her profession and her instinctive need to provide a home environment for her 10-year-old child and yet escape from her adulterous husband.

They both made the mistake of seeing in the other the means of escape from their individual predicaments, and possibly each led the other to believe this to be so. In the case of Sheila, the deep maternal instinct to see a 'nest' in which to rear her remaining child overrode her normally highly intelligent and analytical mind. In the case of Arthur, his dormant, but potentially strong sexual need was soon gratified in a clandestine affair. Clandestine maybe, had it not been for a well placed bath cap discovered in their bathroom during Arthur's first wife's absence! Had it not been for this and the ensuing storm, Arthur's affair would without a doubt have blown itself out. As it was he was trapped, with dire consequences for all, except that Sheila achieved her objective of a 'nest' in which to bring up her fledgling, after which Arthur had served his purpose.

The marriage ('You're committed to marrying me, having shared my bed.') lasted some ten years. Not an ideal match, I often thought, with such different personalities with so little in common, but somehow they each seemed to be resigned to their individual roles going their separate ways, but as long as they were seen apart each one had a personality which gave the superficial impression of an acceptable late-middle-age marriage. Sheila was much more intelligent than Arthur, but not making any demands other than material requirements from time to time. The fledgling, who had the appropriate nickname of 'cuckoo', proved to be as academically gifted as her mother and matured into an attractive young woman. She showed a natural physical liking for her stepfather, probably because she felt safe.

At about the same time as the fledgling showed signs of leaving the nest her mother became increasingly distant and critical of her temporary husband (for that is what events were to make him) and scathing about his occasional friendly advances.

An example of the gathering storm was shown by Arthur's recounting of one holiday incident!

"We went on holiday to South America." (Surprisingly they 'travelled well' together.) "We were in a very deserted part of the country prone to earthquakes.

"After a particularly tedious and dusty journey across the Patagonian desert we arrived at a collection of huts which passed for the local hotel. I collapsed on to a bunk and Sheila repaired to the loo, at that moment there was a noticeable earth tremor and Sheila shouted in an exasperated voice, "And *now* what do you want?" But, as I have said, we somehow managed to coexist on a non-emotional plane."

One day I was called in to see Sheila and was concerned at how languid she had become. Normally a keen gardener, she admitted that she simply could not summon any interest in anything. More as an excuse to give me time to think I took her blood pressure and, to my horror, found that it was so high as to be nearly off the scale. I sent her for investigations which revealed a benign tumour of her parathyroid glands. She was admitted quickly to hospital and, after surgery, she made an uneventful recovery.

This event was to prove the precipitant factor in the breakdown of the marriage, as this type of tumour can often lead to para-psychiatric symptoms, and so it was to prove.

Arthur resumes his story,

"My wife was suffering from bouts of depression which I coped with as best I could. She was an avid reader, but still recovering from her operation, and we spent most evenings sitting on either side of a roaring log fire. I would study her closely; you cannot live closely with someone without acquiring an affection for them, and I had a genuine desire for her complete recovery. After all, we were getting on in years (I was in my 60s), and whatever the reasons for coming together, I loved my home and wished for Sheila to share these creature comforts.

"Suddenly, one evening, sitting on opposite sides of the fire as usual in our large sitting room, she snapped the book which she was reading shut and announced, "We have decided that we are no longer going to live together." I remonstrated at this unilateral decision, but fear gripped my heart, for I knew she was a single-minded and determined lady.

"However, she repeated this statement over several weeks, in spite of my saying it was not my wish that we should part, and eventually she seemed so determined that she put it in writing. After many painful weeks I realised that I was losing the battle for our joint destiny and went to see our solicitor for advice."

It was at about this time that Arthur came for a consultation, for he had developed a rash on one side of his chest. It was an easy diagnosis to make, for he had developed herpes zoster (or shingles), a condition often associated with worry or when bodily resistance is low due to anxiety.

At this time, too, solicitors were involved, and because of the need to see Arthur regularly I had a ringside seat.

As both Arthur and Sheila were being treated by me at this time, I was saddened to watch the tragedy unfold. Sheila was adamant that she 'wanted out', whilst I watched helplessly as Arthur began to lose weight. On many occasions I found him weeping silently, apparently no more able to change his developing destiny than a bullock going to slaughter. Thus an uncomfortable situation proceeded to unfold.

Sheila maintained a totally unemotional exterior and at our meetings she might have been arranging her next holiday for all the concern she displayed.

Arthur takes up the story,

"Sheila soon found a solicitor, and I was fortunate in finding a solicitor who quickly became a friend, and so, over the next trying six months, a bitter legal battle got under way.

"A ridiculous situation arose when Sheila and I (when I managed to remain composed) resumed our usual cool relationship, and would open our post whilst sitting at the breakfast table. Sheila treated the whole developing episode as she might a court case. I became exasperated at the futility of it all when we might have been much more constructive if we had tried to talk about things together.

"Each morning, reviewing our respective posts, I felt as though I was participating in a game of poker, each of us trying, whilst maintaining our civility, to guess what the other held in his or her hand.

"Finally, I had had enough and announced that I was going to short-circuit the whole absurd charade and phone her solicitor, which I did in Sheila's presence. I felt that she would like to have reported me to the Bar Council!

"Eventually her solicitor agreed to speak to me, although I could sense the disappointment in his voice, as, until that moment, his fees were accumulating nicely. I explained that my wife had not been well and that I feared for her health, suggesting that we should meet and bridge the remaining small financial difference between us.

"Reluctantly, I sensed, he agreed, and he came to the house. Just as well, as it turned out, as a QC was being lined up by the 'opposition' to do battle!

"When he arrived, I invited him to take his solicitor's hat off and come for a walk round the garden. I was pleasantly surprised to find an apparently normal human being and we had little difficulty in arriving at a rational solution when I pointed out that I feared for my wife's health and well-being. I then suggested that he replaced his solicitor's hat before going into the house where he met Sheila.

"I was slightly disappointed to hear him tell her that 'your husband has agreed to all our demands'. The final hurt came when Sheila suggested that it 'might be better if you were to find a home outside Gloucestershire'!

"I still do not know what my offence was, calling for my removal from the county I had come to regard as home, but such was my distress that I did. I moved to a flat in another county, feeling very lonely and sorry for myself."

This must be a common enough story, and though I have no solution, I would make one observation and a critical one. I am bound to deplore the way in which some members of the legal profession encourage animosity between parties, rising to mutual hate, when instead conciliation should surely be the primary consideration. Perhaps the explanation is to be found in the chapter on argentosis?

Chapter Thirteen

AIDS

In this section I am grateful to Mr Peter Fraser-Mackenzie, the AIDS control co-ordinator to the Commercial Farmers' Union of Zimbabwe, for his help and for providing figures relating to AIDS in Africa.

AIDS has been singled out for special mention because, unlike some of the other 'natural' threats which are still in the earlier stages of their evolution, AIDS has already established its position as a major killer and even a threat to the human species, and is likely to remain so.

1) AIDS is pandemic and constitutes the most serious threat to the survival of the human race that has ever been encountered. This notwithstanding an American report stating that the disease will be confined in that country to those sectors of the community 'at special risk', i.e., homosexuals and drug users. In the light of the already spreading and rising incidence of heterosexual HIV positive cases this is considered an irresponsible conclusion and likely to put people off their guard.

2) It is still, after some fifteen years, only at the beginning of its invariably fatal destructive cycle.

3) No cure or vaccine is likely in the foreseeable future. Looking further ahead, retroviruses offer some hope for vaccine development, but nothing is likely to materialise before the next millennium.

4) It is likely to decimate whole continents in the next ten to twenty years. Principally Third World countries.

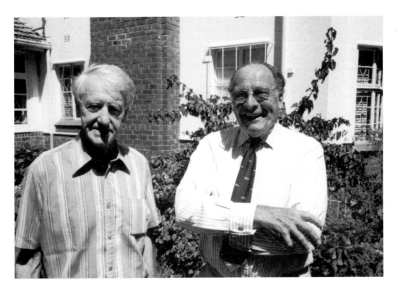

Author *(right)* with previous Prime Minister of Southern
Rhodesia, Mr. Ian Smith.

Author.

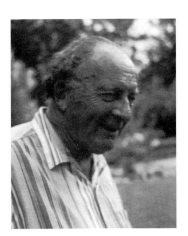

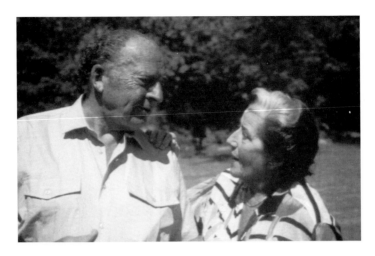

Author with his wife.

The author listens intently to his old chief as he did when he was House Physician in 1944.

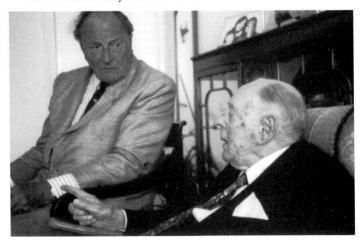

Brief History

There is considerable controversy over the origin and timing of the illness which has come to be known in the public mind as AIDS. It came to the notice of the general public in the early 80s, when a mysterious debilitating illness, which turned out in many cases to be fatal, struck in California.

It was initially not associated with a similar fatal illness which had been present in Africa for a long time, and which was known there as Slim's Disease, on account of the progressive wasting leading to death.

AIDS (or Acquired Immune Deficiency Syndrome) lies dormant for many years, during which time the victim appears to be in good health, but is HIV positive and is highly infectious to others with whom he might come into intimate contact. Although outwardly healthy, his fate is sealed as soon as he becomes HIV positive which, in itself, might not be detectable in tests for up to 90 days after contracting the condition.

He (or she, for both sexes are equally susceptible from heterosexual contact), will surely die within a period of between one to eight years. Congenitally infected babies die within 18 months.

In the early years after the disease was recognised the victims were either:

a)   Intravenous drug users (using infected needles).

b)   Male homosexuals.

c)   Infected by blood transfusions which had not been screened for the virus, and therefore haemophiliacs who required multiple transfusions were highly at risk.

d)   To these three groups must be added a fourth, which is rapidly outnumbering the other three other groups put together, certainly in Africa, and that is heterosexuals with a particular tendency to promiscuity. The same applies to any Third World country, but owing to a misguided policy of nationally denying the existence of the disease in many countries, figures have not been compiled, and the disease is flourishing but unrecognised.

The most important factors facilitating the spread of the disease are:

1) The ability of the virus to *change* its characteristics repeatedly, and so nullify all attempts to halt its proliferation. By 1995 there were eight different identifiable strains of the virus. The first evidence of a single person becoming infected by two different strains of the virus playing 'cupid' was announced in 1995, when the two strains merged to give rise to a new third strain in the host.

2) Man's self-damning characteristic of *promiscuity* which is in direct proportion to:

3) *Mobility*. Thus, the number of 'seat miles' available by road, sea or air in a country has a direct bearing on the morbidity and spread of the virus. The 'return ticket syndrome' ensures that the virus is passed on to the partner remaining at home.

This is reflected in the Zimbabwe figures of AIDS cases, which would indicate that, whilst the overall morbidity of those being HIV positive is 15–20% of the whole population, this figure varies widely from an estimated 17% of the farm populations (low mobility), 22% for rural adults, 27% for urban adults and 35% of skilled workers (affluence plays a part here). Finally, the uniformed (armed services) group 'are unlikely to be less than 50% positive', soldiers on detached duty in Mozambique being highest at risk.

4) The *long incubation* period (seven to eight years or even longer) to the terminal symptoms, during which the victim is apparently healthy, and, more important, virile, though highly infectious.

5) The severe *constrictions on routine testing* for the virus imposed on medical workers makes for difficulty in compiling reliable statistics, as well as encouraging 'innocent' transmission of the disease. As the result, estimates of the morbidity of the disease have always understated the figures, which have required repeated upward revisions.

The only statistics are those for deaths from AIDS. Because of the long lead-in before fully blown AIDS develops, including death, any statistics relating to HIV positive are highly misleading as to the real position, and understate dramatically.

6) *Lack of public awareness.* Despite periodic publicity about AIDS, a time is reached when, like any public health warning, the law of diminishing returns comes into play, reinforced by a lack of tangible evidence of the presence of the disease which reinforces the complacency. This is linked to:

7) *It can't happen to me* syndrome, especially when a person is confronted with a tempting and superficially attractive situation.

Notwithstanding the above, there is some evidence of a shift, however small, in habits. There appears to be less promiscuity and an increasing use of condoms due to some awareness, which, however vague, is likely to be taking place amongst those most at risk. The most important factor to recall is that, whatever happens, there are eight years of irrevocable deaths already in the pipeline.

It is estimated that by the year 2000 there will be 40 million people in the world who are already HIV positive.

The World Health Organisation has announced that, in 1994, four million new HIV positive cases were identified, more than all the new cases identified in the 1980s. Dr Jonathan Mann, professor of Epidemiology at Harvard, stated, "The worst is yet to come, and the campaign against AIDS is losing its impetus."

A disturbing trend in California is that the number of new cases, having fallen after the early warnings were given, has now climbed again to its original alarming levels.

Depopulation

When the incidence of HIV positive reaches somewhere between 18–25% of the inhabitants of a country, which is the probability in many African countries before the end of the decade, the rate of new infections is likely to stabilise. At the same time, the population also stabilises rather than continues to increase. A significant reduction in population is unlikely to take place until nearly 50% of the adult population has become infected.

However, severe disruption of the economy and social structure will already have occurred, because the productive section of the population will, for practical purposes, have been eliminated. It has been estimated that 60% of the 25–29-year-old females in Zimbabwe would have become infected by mid 1995, and these figures may well be exceeded in certain other African countries. This will result in one million orphans being created at the same time, with a dire shortage of grandparents to look after them.

It does not call for much imagination to conclude that a critical economic scenario is about to envelop many African countries, and probably much of Asia also, with the gross depletion of the working population. The resulting poverty will lead increasingly to females 'selling' their bodies, leading to an over-supply and thus exacerbating the spread of the disease to the remaining, but dwindling numbers of healthy, maturing males. This will take place all within the next few years, and certainly by the turn of the century in sub-Sahara Africa.

The Next Step – Restocking The World?

Starting with sub-Sahara Africa in the early part of the 21st century, and assuming that Europe and the Western world has not totally succumbed to the AIDS devastation, the need and opportunity to restock Africa will arise.

Africa will lie devastated but potentially one of the richest continents in the world in terms of natural wealth, minerals, energy sources, and productive climate, lacking for nothing except the ingenuity of modern man. A tempting prize indeed, but for whom?

America and Europe will be struggling with their own peculiar economic and health problems, not helped by internal political strife as capitalism exhausts itself. Simultaneously, the Western world will be striving to meet the ever-demanding needs of the United Nations in that body's efforts to contain the minor wars and threats to wreck civilisation.

In this world of unrest the dying embers of black Africa, its peoples bewildered at the decimation which has engulfed them, will be struggling in their death throes like flies sprayed with insecticide. The depopulated continent will beckon, waiting to be seized and recolonised, but by whom, and who would dare to risk becoming contaminated by the diseased population?

One contender is already flexing her muscles: China! For centuries, China has been biding her time, but her moment may well be nigh. In 1997 she acquired a 'lung' or gateway to the world through Hong Kong. Through Hong Kong, China stands to learn both the benefits to be derived from capitalism as well as its dangers. Her population is numerous enough to be expendable should the need arise, and her technological advance is becoming impressive. She has one billion workers accustomed to work for a dollar an hour and has already tested the climate of Africa.

In recent commercial ventures in Africa, when several thousand Chinese have been sent to that continent they have kept very much to themselves and avoided fraternisation; there were no Sino-African children left behind. That amounts to the equivalent of a vaccine against the AIDS virus. Given a Chinese colonisation of Africa, how would the rest of the world stand for the future?

Conclusion

In the meantime, to understand how the distribution of AIDS might develop in the Western world, we should take heed of the studies undertaken in Zimbabwe where substantial inroads into the heterosexual population have been made. In particular, it should be noted that a forecast for 1995 showed:

- 18% of the total population will be HIV positive and will therefore die within 4–8 years.
- 33% of the population aged 15–50 will be similarly infected and will also die within 4–8 years.
- 60% of the females aged 25–29 will be infected and die within 4–8 years.
- Females are more prone to becoming infected than males.

AIDS – Update (1997)

Since the World Health Organisation compiled the figures four years ago, there are some signs that the nature of the disease has marginally modified its characteristics. There has been a marked shift towards heterosexual infections – especially in Third World countries, and also some evidence of autoimmunity, although it is too early to attach much significance to this. The latest statistical news from the WHO is that:

- There is a total of 22 million HIV positive cases in the world.

- Two-thirds of these are in sub-Sahara Africa.
- 1.5 million deaths from AIDS have taken place.
- But – the most serious aspect – there have been 2.5 million new cases of infection during the last year.

Moreover, the statistical sources of these figures are notoriously unreliable, so there is no room for complacency.

Meanwhile, the only way of combating AIDS lies primarily through education and thereby changing sexual habits to monosex or safe sex.

The maxim should be – there are no second chances!

The words of Marie Stopes are relevant if slightly out of context: 'The best form of contraception is 'NO'!'

The stigma attached to AIDS must be removed. The Princess of Wales did much to this end.

The retrograde rule that doesn't allow patients to be tested for AIDS without their permission should be abolished, for this only serves to drive the disease underground. This rule applies to no other illness and it is surely contrary to all one's medical training to single out one particular illness for special guidelines. Testing for AIDS should be parcelled with any routine investigatory procedure. The fact that it is a fatal illness does not isolate it in any way from any other fatal illness, and the justification of its being a 'social' illness with stigma attached is overruled in the general interest of the public at large, not to mention the very survival of the human race.

Indeed it is the policy of certain airlines to test all pilots for the disease as a routine procedure, because of the risk of dementia associated with the illness.

Complacency is the greatest ally that viruses have. A cunning fox will jump into the chicken coop and then sit quietly while the hens complacently settle down again so that they can be picked off one by one at the fox's will; so it is with the AIDS virus.

By November 1994, new cases of HIV positive in San Francisco were again up to the levels they were at when the virus was first discovered, i.e., safe sex is now being ignored.

Though too early to be more than a hope, or even a wish, there are grounds for believing that AIDS might – and only might – burn itself out, as myxomatosis did for rabbits. Meanwhile though, there is evidence indicating that the virus is becoming more virulent, and the interval between infection and death is shortening.

Notwithstanding all this gloom and doom, life is precious and its preservation is a deeply ingrained instinct throughout the animal kingdom and, in the case of *Homo sapiens*, not confined to one's own life, but to those of others as well.

Whilst we ponder on the greater issues relating to man's future the main task of living today still has to be coped with. Those aches and pains and what to do with them. Well, spare-part surgery is increasingly available, advancing in line with computer-provided facilities and techniques. Even 'heroic surgical procedures' are widely available, to the delight of the media, who are always on the lookout for anything unusual, and always providing that the increasing army of bureaucrats is willing to authorise payment for it.

Increasing financial constraints are progressively clouding the wider field of medicine, for treatments are becoming more expensive, and the resources to provide for the more complex arrangements become more scarce. Is this another version of argentosis?

The courts struck a blow for medicine in making it known that, in their view, any decision on the 'allocation of available resources' is not a legal matter, but one to be decided by the medical profession (this was in relation to the treatment of a child with leukaemia). This ruling has important implications for how the needs of the elderly should be catered for. As a result of this ruling it would seem rational and effective to shift the responsibility for caring for the elderly progressively from social services to being a medical responsibility, and thus eliminate what is becoming an increasingly expensive grey zone.

Although nature carries out routine replacements on most body cells, the exception is the brain, where, from the earliest days of life, only steady deterioration takes place. As cells die they are not replaced, which, as everyone of middle age or older knows only too well, means that names, facts and other simple mental tasks become elusive and irretrievable. To repeat (deliberately, lest you forget): in the case of the brain, it is downhill all the way from birth, with the cells gradually but irrevocably dying without being replaced. The apparent increase in mental performance in the first half of life is due solely to better utilisation of what remains of the diminishing brain. It is like a torch whose battery is steadily running down, but which, providing the bulb is replaced occasionally and the parts kept clean, should give adequate service until near the end.

I pondered on this thought when I was spending a few days on a fruit farm in Zimbabwe.

As I watched the steady stream of apples, some 1,000,000 a year, rolling down a conveyor belt, I reflected that I might well be watching a nation of humans going through life. Starting with the smallest, which fell through onto one of six sizing apertures, leaving the largest to avoid selection until the end of the line, by which time their numbers had been severely pruned, the clatter of the machinery, coupled with the steady stream of fruit passing in front of my eyes, had a mesmerising effect. Various shapes and sizes streamed past, some with green skins, some red, some slightly bruised, the latter being promptly removed by one of the African girls watching for sub-standard fruit. It was similar to standing on an escalator at a London Underground station watching passengers being carried to their destinations.

As the smaller apples fell through the sorting holes, the remainder continued in diminishing numbers, leaving the largest to progress to the final belt, which delivered them into a box marked 'Most Prime', and eventually the now-empty conveyor belt continued into a black hole.

Suddenly the metaphor dawned on me: humans are but apples!

I walked from the grading shed through one of the many orchards where the trees were nurtured (the nursery), treated with insecticides (vaccinated), the blossom fertilised by bees kept specially for this purpose, and any windfalls discarded (neo-natal mortality).

Once picked from the trees, the ultimate fate of each apple is predetermined. Up to a point, so is our future, though we have an element of influence over whether we reach the 'prime grade'.

Enjoy your apples. So you might ask, or indeed desire, 'Why can't I live for well over a hundred more years, enjoy the fruits of my labours, and see how things develop?' Why not indeed? Dr Nat Armstrong has not only managed it, but has retained all his mental faculties in first-class order (see frontispiece.)

Chapter Fourteen
Coronary Thrombosis.

Heart Attack

The term 'heart attack' epitomises a dramatic event, an emergency, which it invariably is, requiring quick and precise actions by trained and experienced people. It is, however, an imprecise description, embracing many conditions from transient angina to terminal heart failure. The most important and life-threatening of these is coronary thrombosis, which is but one condition in the broader group of cardiovascular diseases. It is one of the very few medical emergencies and one of four of the most important life-shortening illnesses.

The death rate from coronary heart disease in the United Kingdom is amongst the highest in the world.

- One male in 4 will have a coronary before 65.
- One in 15 will die before 65 – a total of 50,000 a year.
- 20% of these deaths are smoking-related.
- 40,000 females will die each year from a coronary. It is the second commonest cause of death in females after cancer.
- One in three coronary attacks are 'silent' and not recognised at the time.

As smoking is becoming less common in the developed countries, at least amongst middle-aged and older people (the group most likely to be attacked), so the incidence of coronary attacks is falling, especially in North America. There, deaths from coronaries have dropped from a peak in 1960 of 236 per 100,000 to 115 in 1988, i.e., more than halved. However, this encouraging trend may well be reversed as the younger new smokers continue to indulge their killing habits as they mature into middle age.

Coronary's first cousin, angina, often a precursor of a coronary, is also linked to smoking. For every death from coronary thrombosis there are fifteen angina sufferers, many of whom will be called by the grim reaper in due course.

What is coronary thrombosis? To understand how to avoid it we need to have some working knowledge of what it is all about.

In order to carry out its principal function of pumping blood around the body, the heart muscles (there are four separate chambers in the heart) need a continuous and adequate supply of oxygen, like any other working muscle. This oxygen is supplied by the four coronary arteries, which embrace the outside of the heart muscle chambers. If they become 'furred up' then the heart muscle becomes starved of oxygen and, like cramp in the leg, pain occurs. If a portion of the artery becomes totally blocked, perhaps by a clot forming, then that part of the muscle supplied by the artery will eventually die and be replaced by scar tissue, which is termed a myocardial infarct, and will show up on an electrocardiograph (ECG), as the scar tissue will not conduct the electrical impulse vital to the effective functioning of the heart as an organ.

The victim may not be aware that he has suffered a heart attack and approximately one third all coronaries are symptomless and only discovered at an autopsy or an ECG. All that the victim may be aware of is that (s)he is short of breath.

If the coronary arteries become narrowed without being blocked, then the condition of angina will occur, causing chest pain, often extending down the left arm, especially on exertion or under stress. This condition causes considerable discomfort and even distress, and may well precipitate a coronary unless heeded and relieved by appropriate treatment, such as rest and glycerol trinitrite inhalants (TNT capsules).

Although an ECG will reveal if a patient has had a coronary at some time in his life, it is not possible to say with certainty whether he is going to have one. Indeed, I well recall visiting an eminent physician in Leeds for the purpose of obtaining a medical report for life insurance purposes. Ominously, I reflected, his consulting rooms were on the fourth floor without a lift, and on struggling, gasping, to the top, I found my physician waiting, having watched me struggling up the stairs.

While I regained my breath he beckoned me to sit down, meanwhile filling out some forms. After some time he said,

"Well, that's most of the medical examination completed, manipulating the stairs!" After a few more cursory probings he completed his form filling, and said, "Had an embarrassment the other week; chap like yourself, looked fit, though I did have some misgivings about his weight. The ECG was normal, so I bade him farewell and completed his insurance proposal form. Just as I was about to sign it my nurse came in, clearly agitated. "That patient of yours, Doctor, he has just collapsed as he was getting into a taxi in the street; dead, I'm afraid."" The physician put down his pen. "What would you have done? Signed him as a normal risk?"

I didn't reply, nor will I divulge what that physician did, but what would you have done?

A series of post-mortems on young service pilots killed in air crashes revealed that 'furring up' (arteriosclerosis) was present in a significant proportion of their coronary arteries. Before considering which factors should be studied when considering how to prevent a coronary, it cannot be emphasised too strongly the part which smoking plays, not only in cardiovascular disease as a whole, but in the foreshortening of life in general not only for the smokers themselves, but for those who have the misfortune to live in close proximity to smokers.

It used to be thought that smoking was something that would kill in old age; that is simply not so. Lung cancer is not the only significant smoking risk, there are at least twenty other diseases. Half of the victims will die in middle age, losing some twenty-four years of normal, useful life, and those who survive into old age will forfeit eight years.

If, as a smoker, you have an interest as to how you might finish (be finished, if you prefer to have it put that way): of 1000 smokers, it has been shown that one will be murdered, 6 will die in road accidents, and 300 from a tobacco-related death. Of greatest importance, however, it will be in all probability an earlier death.

I am frequently asked if I have ever smoked; the simple answer is, 'Of course, when I was young, and not particularly health conscious'. In the early 1950s, before the dangers from smoking had been recognised, I used to sit on a certain committee on which an eminent statistician, Sir Austin Bradford Hill, also sat. One day, he said he felt there was surely a link between smoking and lung cancer, but was not certain how to prove it. It was suggested, seeing that the room was full of smoke, that perhaps he might conduct a study amongst the medical profession, and that is exactly what happened. Some months later I was enjoying my occasional after-breakfast cigarette when the morning post arrived, containing a formal letter from Bradford Hill's department at the London School of Hygiene and Tropical Medicine enquiring whether I would be prepared to be enlisted in a survey on smokers. I happily complied, filling in the questionnaire as to how many cigarettes I smoked, inhaling habits and so forth.

Two years later, still smoking, though by now I had developed a troublesome cough, came the follow-up questionnaire, which commenced 'Dear Doctor, If you are still alive...'

I have not smoked since! I did, however, participate in one further trial by Bradford Hill relating to the role of aspirin in coronaries, and so far am glad to report that I survived that one too! (Half an aspirin, taken daily, significantly reduces the risk of a heart attack.)

Causes of death are not as important as the age at which those causes occur, for diseases which happen early in life are responsible for 'lost years' of life. Viewed in this way (see also Chapter Ten), coronary heart disease poses a major threat to family happiness, for life-depriving fatal coronaries tend all too frequently to come in a person's 40s, and as they can to a considerable degree be prevented, then this form of death must be placed into the 'voluntary' death category (along with the three other common life-depriving illnesses, i.e., road traffic accidents, some forms of cancer, and suicides).

How, then, can one assess whether one is at risk from coronary thrombosis and what might one do about it?

There are six major and several minor factors to be considered. Of the six major factors only one is beyond your control – your genes.

1. Hereditary

If a very close relation (father, mother, brother) has died or has suffered a major coronary before the age of 55, count 3 points for each victim. If it is a more remote relative (uncle, aunt, grandparent) who has suffered a major coronary before the age of 50, count 2 points for each one.

2. Smoking

If you have smoked more that 5 cigarettes a day in the last year, 10 in either of the previous 2 years, 20 in any of the previous 3 years, count 1 point for each year, multiplied by each excess factor for that year (i.e., for 5 x 1, for 10 x 2, for 20 x 4, if this is what you have smoked in the last year).

For example, if you haven't smoked for a year, but smoked 20 cigarettes in each of the previous 4 years, then score $2+2+1+1=6$.

3. Overweight

This has to be age-related, and to experience a modest 'age weight gain' is not necessarily life-threatening, but may be if accompanied by a significant rise in blood pressure. Providing that one is within a 'normal' shape parameter at the age of 21 (standard weight charts are useful guides, but no more), then a 10% weight gain spread evenly over the next 30 years and a further 5% over the following 20 years should not give cause for draconian dietetic measures. It should still be compatible with a healthy lifestyle as well as with an ability to get reasonable wear from one's wardrobe without regular adjustments from one's tailor. Any sudden diversion from these guidelines should be addressed severely however. It should also be remembered that it might be equally injurious to health to be underweight as to be overweight.

Score half a point for each pound over a straight line 'gain' for each year outside the above guidelines. A score in excess of 10 should be cause for reflection.

4. Hypertension

Raised blood pressure is often a direct consequence of being overweight and should be assessed together with weight rather than in isolation, so that the above guidelines for weight may be more significant and pruned accordingly. There are two measurements by which blood pressure is assessed.

The higher of the two readings (systolic) is the more variable, and, at least in part, is a measure of the suppleness of the arteries. It will also vary with stress, exercise, and excitement. As a rough guide, it is normal if it measures 100 millimetres of mercury plus your age.

The second reading (diastolic) is lower than the first, and reflects the pressure left in your arteries whilst the heart pump is refilling. It reflects the suppleness of your arteries. Conversely, one might compare the hardness of a hosepipe which has spent the summer exposed to the sun.

The diastolic pressure is much less variable from day to day and is therefore the more significant as an underlying measure of health. The principal danger from abnormally raised blood pressure is that either a clot may form, or, more significantly, a blood vessel may actually burst like an over-inflated car tyre, usually with dire consequences. The good news is that high blood pressure more often than not responds to appropriate treatment. It cannot be stressed too strongly that smoking damages the blood vessels, making them weaker and more prone to both clotting and bursting.

5. Exercise

We should consider a simple analogy: if a new car has its engine started at the beginning of a day, and is then left in its garage to continue ticking over at minimum revolutions, what would be the likelihood of that car still running by the end of three days? The chances are that the plugs might well be 'sooted up'. And so with an otherwise healthy human. For a young to middle-aged person a totally sedentary life is both physiologically and psychologically most unhealthy. Muscle tone is lost and muscles become flabby, and even bowel habits become sedentary, not to mention the state of the heart and circulatory system.

As a guideline, even a moderate amount of exercise, sufficient to make you sweat, will go a long way to creating normal health. Such a guideline should go a long way towards reducing the risk of a coronary, possibly by 25%.

Up to the age of 35, score 2 points for each (of 4) days in a week when this yardstick is not reached, and similarly one point between the age of 35 and 60.

After the age of 60, exercise is not so essential though psychologically (as in golf) it may well be beneficial.

Surprisingly, there is no evidence to suggest that golfers have any significant immunity from cardiovascular disease, other than the controversial benefit derived at the 19th hole. The significance of this may lie in the fact that golf does not qualify as exercise as defined above.

Even the reverse may be true in that it would appear that golfers are more prone to accidents and joint problems.

One final warning: once past 50 years of age, be your age! Avoid jogging. More sudden deaths occur whilst jogging than any other sport, with the possible exception of squash. Have you ever seen a 'happy jogger', or even had a smile from one? I suspect that they are anticipating a sudden end, and I always avoid them like the plague.

Many people say that exercise is essential for good health (health and fitness are not synonymous). Health is consistent with 'being well', being free from illness, and is not necessarily brought about by exercise, so much as by lifestyle.

Fitness is frequently, but not necessarily brought about by exercise. It can be psychological in form, and may be mental with minimum physical involvement, such as being fit to play a musical instrument, but essentially it implies fitness for a purpose, rather than good health.

Thus it is tempting to conclude that exercise is not essential at all, but that would be tempting fate, even though human beings can be confined in small areas for extended periods, as in prison.

How beneficial, if not essential, is exercise for health, even important, in order to carry out a function, physical or mental? 'Limited' may well be the truthful answer.

As the amount of exercise increases, so does the psychological benefit which can be derived, leading to a feeling of well-being – an important constituent of a good life.

On the other hand, should you feel disinclined to take exercise, it does not follow that you must make an early reservation in the nearest four-star cemetery. Very much the reverse, for you may well have the final laugh over your frenetically exercising mentors, and this becomes more so with advancing years, leading into late middle age. The facts do not paint a reassuring story:

Sudden exercise-related deaths in the United Kingdom, 1978-1987:

SPORT	AVERAGE AGE & RANGE	NUMBER OF DEATHS
Squash	44 (22–70)	126
Swimming	53 (14–84)	56
Soccer	42 (17–61)	53
Running	37 (11–71)	39
Badminton	49 (27–82)	26
Rugby	30 (15–52)	14
Other Sports	Not available	37

These frenetic exercisers, whilst they may enjoy a very real sense of personal well-being and self-satisfaction, as long as they survive, out of all proportion to the physical benefit, sometimes take on predatory characteristics. These are accompanied by an air of self-righteousness and a tendency to proselytise perfectly content people; prising them out of their chairs to a less comfortable environment, and even, possibly, a more dangerous one.

To err on the safe side, assuming you want to live a little longer, I would counsel, for those in middle age:

1) No more exercise than you feel inclined to take.

2) Be very wary of taking up any exercise too enthusiastically, unless you are used to it.

For those under 45, however, I would recommend, as an anti-coronary measure, considering the following:

Increase your pulse rate by 20% over your 'resting' pulse rate for 20 minutes 4-7 days a week by non-emotional means – thus disqualifying, but not excluding sexual activity. A suitable piece of ancillary apparatus would prove a good investment, a dog for example.

Between 45 and 70, the above targets might be progressively reduced by 50% if you choose.

After 70, whilst the same principles apply, avoid any exercise which does not appeal, as by this age the die is more or less cast, (no pun intended).

The three most dangerous sports, that are most likely to precipitate a coronary, are squash, badminton and swimming (as an 'effort'), and the risks increase markedly over the age of 40. There are up to 40 deaths a year on the squash courts in the UK. One third of fatalities on the squash court are known to have had prior heart conditions.

For those still determined to play, say, squash, ask yourself a few questions. If the answer is 'yes' to any of the following, pause and reflect, and consider having a simple medical examination before playing. Answering yes to two should be mandatory.

Do you answer 'yes' to any of the following?

1) Over 60?

2) Any chest pains?

3) Do you get short of breath or have dizzy spells after exercise?

4) Are you diabetic?

5) Do you suffer from angina or any heart condition? (Or have you had heart surgery?)

6) Any history of raised blood pressure?

7) Do you smoke?

8) Had any black outs?

The squash rackets association's maxim is: 'Get fit to play squash. Don't play to get fit'.

Post script: To doubters who still believe that daily exercise is essential, there is no evidence to indicate that airline pilots, who lead a very sedentary life, have a reduced expectation of life, and they might be thought to follow a very unhealthy lifestyle:

i) Sleeping/resting at irregular times, constantly transgressing time zones.

ii) Irregular attention to bodily needs – food, bowels.

iii) Long periods of bodily and mental inactivity, with accompanying stress due to boredom, with added stress potential from the unexpected.

iv) Short bursts of intense activity.

v) Fluctuating exposures to changing environmental pressure and temperatures.

vi) Exposure to above normal radiation levels.

vii) Minimal opportunities for exercise.

Though it cannot be denied that exercise has an important part to play in the promotion of well-being, it is equally prudent to repeat the warning that exercise is not without risk, in the same way as taking to the air is, so that its place in the actual prolongation of life is debatable.   As has been observed, jogging is a common, if somewhat artificial way of indulging in exercise, but I have always been somewhat discouraged from taking it up by the all too frequent sudden deaths which seem to overtake those who are to be seen puffing round our public parks and lanes.

There was some correspondence a few years ago on the merits of exercise, in the *British Medical Journal*, which disclosed some disquieting facts on the risks appertaining to playing sports in general.   One letter read:

> *500 deaths have occurred in accidents during sports and leisure activities in the last five reported years, as well as other deaths during exercise from pre-existing disease.*
>
> *Last Saturday, I played cricket in a team without its regular wicket keeper, who was in hospital recovering from a heart attack that had occurred during a game of squash, against a team missing a player who had died after being struck by lightning whilst playing golf.*

I mused that the benefits of sport are not as clear cut as some might have us believe.

> *Furthermore, [the letter continued] in 1988, half a million people aged sixteen and over, and 200,000 children attended accident and emergency departments in the United Kingdom after sports accidents.   From these small numbers it has been officially estimated that there were one and a half million exercise-related injuries needing contact with a doctor, resulting in five and a half million days lost from work (1988). Subsequent figures, not yet published, would seem to indicate that even these official figures underestimate*

*the problem. Thus, whilst exercise indisputably confers
health benefits, it also incurs substantial health costs.*

Thinking this publication might be a hoax, I wrote to the author, Jon Nicoll, at Sheffield Medical School, who assured me that his information was taken from published figures, and he admitted that he was searching for an alternative to exercise as a means of keeping in good health – 'If you can find such a solution, you have certainly hit the jackpot'. The debate continues, but my considered advice would be for everyone to follow his own inclination regarding exercise and keep smiling (which of course excludes jogging!)!

Put in quantitative cost terms, figures released by the Sports Council in 1993 calculate that each year 19 million sports injuries cost £0.5 billion in treatment and days lost from work. Also that nearly half of 16–45 year olds play sport at least once a month, and their injuries to joints, bones, soft tissues and faces cost some £240 million to be treated.

It might be prudent to issue a 'death warning' with every pair of running shoes sold, and maybe to install a life insurance machine on the first tee at golf clubs, similar to those (occasionally) available at airports. Come to think of it, flags at golf clubs do seem to fly at half mast on a suspiciously frequent number of days. At the risk of alienating my numerous golfing friends, I have been unable to find any evidence that the playing of golf extends one's life expectancy.

Cholesterol

This is controversial, and the craze to avoid animal fats and stay with polyunsaturated fatty acids in one's diet waxes and wanes according to the current fashion. The whole subject of body lipids, of which cholesterol is arguably the most important, fills many pages in any respectable medical textbook, but whether one is any healthier for reading is not certain. That lipids play a major part in laying down fat on the walls of selective arteries is not in doubt, and if one is in danger of having a coronary or stroke on other grounds, then one should without doubt take heed and take action as required.

Moreover, it can be reassuring, if only because it is one of the few clinical tests that can be done on oneself by buying the apparatus for a few pounds from a chemist.

Recent research would seem to indicate that the importance of raised blood cholesterol decreases with age, being important in middle age when coronaries are more likely to occur, and less important the older one becomes and the more one moves out of the acute danger zone.

For a point count, collect 3 points for a high reading between 40 and 55, 2 points for a reading between 55 and 70, and one point thereafter.

After 80, if you are still enjoying life it is probably because you enjoy whatever food comes your way including all farm products. Keep going!

For a quick, simple self-assessment: if you are adversely affected by 2 or more of the above 6 factors, then rearrange your lifestyle to eradicate the adverse factors. Otherwise, 'Be Prepared...'

Summary – How to Avoid a Heart Attack:

A   Analyse the cardiac family history and, if members of your family have suffered coronaries, pay particular attention to the other 5 factors.

B   Don't smoke and avoid close proximity to others who do.

C   Have a pair of bathroom scales, and use them one morning each week; take firm action to control any untoward (2 lb.s or so) gain.

D   Avoid extreme exercise after 40, a 20 minute walk 4 times a week will suffice after 60. NEVER EXERT YOURSELF IN VERY COLD WEATHER (shovelling snow etc.). The cold masks nature's warning signs such as 'overheating', sweating etc.

E   Have your blood pressure checked every three years up to the age of 40, every two years up to 60, and once a year thereafter, more frequently if it rises.

F   Entertain yourself by measuring your own blood cholesterol very occasionally, unless you have cause to be concerned, in which case consult your GP. DIY cholesterol kits can be obtained from your local chemist, but the only safe course– if you are concerned – is to consult your GP.

Chapter Fifteen
Brain Failure – Memory

Two characteristics lie behind the working of the body: chemical reactions and electrical impulses. In this context, human beings can be differentiated from computers, which depend wholly on electrical impulses, which is why computers are devoid of emotion and wisdom.

A cynic might well observe that human beings are increasingly attempting to emulate computers and abdicating what should be human responsibilities in their favour. This might explain why so much is wrong with *Homo sapiens* today. We would do better to continue to concentrate on what we as human beings are good at, such as decision taking and compassion (before we lose it), to name but two characteristics. We have a completely different form of memory from that which a computer has.

How does the human memory, as compared to that of a computer, function? Computer memories, though more extensive than human memories, are straightforward and, as such, are simple. Human memories on the other hand, are complex and prone to failure, and even unreliable.

If I can now remember what I am trying to say, I will try and explain in a simplified way how the human memory functions and how it can be damaged by illness as well as affected by ageing. A little poetic licence will enable the human memory to be understood.

How do we remember, and what can go wrong when memory fails?

Short-Term Memory

Imagine a village pond on a warm, still summer day. Throw a stone into the calm water. The stone will create a ripple of wavelets, each spreading out, rebounding against the banks and leaving an impression on any small floating leaves etc. Soon, the ripples become less well-defined, and after about five minutes, there will be no trace of the impact of the stone, and the pond will resume its placid surface. That is a short-term event, as is short-term memory, the only difference being that in the case of the pond, the ripples are created in water and are visual, whereas the brain's short-term trace is in the form of an electrical impulse capable of carrying visual, auditory, olfactory sensations, pleasure, pain, indeed any sensation that the body can detect. Though vivid in the moment, like a dream, there will be no long-term trace and, unless the impression is transferred to the long term memory bank within a relatively short period of time, it will be lost, just like the ripples on the pond, for ever.

The ability, and the decision to transfer short-term impressions to long-term memory in the form of a permanent record will depend on a number of factors, which can be considered separately, including the ability, and it is this ability which can become impaired by certain lesions and illnesses, including Alzheimer's disease (see Chapter Sixteen).

Long-Term Memory.

Transferring a short-term memory event into a permanent long-term memory recording involves a complex chemical change in the brain cells.

If there is a similar experience already recorded, a 'search' of the memory library will be carried out to try and find it and compare it to the new experience, at which point the person will say (or think), 'Yes, I remember this', be it visual, aural, oral or even olfactory.

If the memory was stored a long time ago, then, like old, faded library books, the chemical shape may well have altered through deterioration; then the memory will search out the nearest 'likeness' for comparison. This explains two phenomena: *déjà vu*, when one gets a feeling that something has happened before, though without the clarity to enable one to be certain, and illusion, such as when revisiting a scene that one hasn't seen for many years (since childhood, for example); the size, shape, even colour of an object may appear to have altered, for example a room might be remembered as smaller than the reality.

This deterioration does not necessarily occur at a uniform rate, for the image may have been laid down in the long-term memory in an imperfect manner, due to, for example, distractions at the time, or lack of concentration. This explains how witnesses in court can be notoriously unreliable unless written notes of the incident were made at the time.

The study of embryology reveals that different parts of the body and their functions develop at different times and rates. Short-term memory ability develops at an earlier age than long-term memory. Only a few early memories of events which happened before the age of four exist. Serious schooling, other than to teach habits, is a waste of time before the age of about five. Child prodigies who can play musical instruments learn more by habit than intellect.

After the age of four or five, memories are laid down at an increasingly faster rate, and those early learnings being received by a virgin memory base are the best learned and the easiest to recall. A practical application of this is that if one learns a skill as a child, such as driving a vehicle, the accident rate as an adult is significantly lower than it would be for a person who doesn't start to drive until later in life. The skill will also be retained longer under conditions of stress, fatigue or sedatives, including alcohol.

Dyslexia

On this subject, I speak with some experience, as at least two of my grandchildren are dyslexic, though in my own case the condition was not recognised as an entity when I was a youngster, and I was simply categorised as 'backward'.

A mild dyslexic has to spend more time and be more thorough than his peers in order to learn any specified task, however, in so doing, he learns things more thoroughly, if painfully, than his fellow pupils. If he can survive his schooling he will emerge in later years as capable, perhaps more so than his 'normal' classmates. The analogy here between the tortoise and the hare would seem appropriate.

The danger is that he may also have developed an inferiority complex and will require a lot of encouragement in the early phases of earning his living. There are compensations, for, as he (or she) grows older, he may also develop a modicum of that valuable but elusive quality: wisdom, and even clarity of thought.

The dyslexic may also develop learning methods which help to overcome the dyslexia itself. By the time he reaches maturity he will have 'caught up' and able to hold his own with a full 'library' of memories.

In certain illnesses, as well as in old age, when searching for something in the long-term memory library the crossmatching can become less reliable, as when brain cells have died, for example. Under these conditions, the failing memory will grasp at anything that has even the remotest resemblance to the current scene, and this leads to mental confusion.

It also has applied practical shortcomings in the practice of routine and continuous skills, such as typing, so that individual groups of letters become reversed or juxtaposed. This happens increasingly frequently with advancing years and is a form of literary 'spoonerism'.

Spoonerism is a verbal example of juxtaposition due to a malfunction in worn brain cells, e.g., 'you have hissed the mystery lesson'.

It also leads to the 'one-track mind' syndrome when only one mental task can be executed at a time; males especially would appear to be disadvantaged. Hurrying downstairs, which calls for a series of complex but familiar repetitive quick muscle movements, activated by a lower centre in the brain, can lead to trouble if the automatic centre 'freezes'.

Certain illnesses destroy brain cells at a faster rate than normal, the pathological rate of destruction seen in Alzheimer's, cerebral atherosclerosis ('hardening of the arteries'), and Parkinson's disease, to name but a few. It is as though specific parts of the brain are being 'dissolved'. But, you may ask, are there ever occasions when extensive damage is done to brain cells but where, miraculously, healing and recovery takes place instead of death?

Yes. One such state is : persistent vegetative state (PVS), if prematurely diagnosed. This condition has, in recent years, attracted increasing attention for two principal reasons:

1)   Increasing standards of nursing care, coupled with technological advances, which enable unconscious persons to be kept alive for longer periods than until recently would have been thought possible.

2) Wider debate about voluntary euthanasia, thus focusing on which circumstances might justify withdrawal of life-support machines when the victim is considered to be brain-dead and when therefore no possibility of recovery exists.

Definition:

PVS must be distinguished from other conditions where consciousness is lost. It is not a brief transitory condition lasting a day or so before a return to a normal conscious state.

In PVS the victim appears to be awake; the eyes are open, although the victim is not aware of anything around him and does not respond to sound, smell or touch. No purposeful movements are made, though the cough reflex remains, as does choking (gagging). The victim appears to go through a form of sleep/waking cycle, some changes in facial expression appear to take place, and the jaw might move.

PVS should be differentiated from.

a) Coma, when the eyes are invariably shut.

b) Certain neurological diseases (multiple sclerosis is one) when there might be total paralysis, but the patient may intimate (through eye movements possibly) that he is aware of his surroundings.

Duration

PVS must persist for approximately six months before being confirmed as a diagnosis, and the patient will have needed artificial (tube) feeding, and will also be incontinent.

Two separate causes can be identified:

a) Traumatic (injury).

b) Non-traumatic (strokes, metabolic upsets, oxygen deprivation, and certain medical conditions, such as a tumour).

Under the heading of 'stroke', one cause might be a fat embolism which is likely to follow a bone injury or an otherwise straightforward operation (usually orthopaedic). In these cases the onset is liable to be sudden, even happening before the patient comes round from an anaesthetic ('He simply won't wake up.').

Whatever the cause, it is a grave life-threatening event and calls for nursing care of a devoted specialised kind, bringing into play techniques and skills which were simply not available thirty years ago.

Prognosis

Reports differ widely. The American Multi-Society Task Force, reviewing their cases, put the three most important factors as *age, cause,* and *duration* of the condition.

The older patients are most at risk, as are those PVS cases brought about by a medical condition, whilst brain injuries stand the best chance of recovering after three months of PVS (one third, albeit with some residual disability).

Of the non-traumatic episodes (strokes etc.), the recovery chances slim down to less than 10% after three months and then with a good deal of residual disability.

The case I describe below is remarkable indeed, especially as the residual disability after recovery is minimal, with regard to the patient's age. Perhaps the most important aspect of the convalescence was the determination with which he recreated and reassembled his memory bank from virtually zero in the early phase of recovering 'consciousness'.

This type of case (PVS) is not to be confused with simple concussion, where the effects are generally short-lived, clearing up in a day or so. The effects in this instance were far-reaching, and lasted in excess of four months.

The spectrum of any brain damage can be likened to the difference between cutting off the power supply to a computer, when the damage may be permanent, and to an electric clock, which can be reset.

Fortunately, the case now described came into the second category, and although four months of his life were irretrievably and permanently lost, the 'clock' was restarted at the current time.

It concerned a man, aged 83, in reasonably good health for his age, although he frankly admitted that his memory, especially for names, was poor. He also had an arthritic hip and had to visit a hospital for a routine hip replacement.

It would be correct, and probably relevant, to say that he was a devout if covert Christian; being covert, he was more devout than an overt Christian might appear to be.

The operation was successful, but he failed to regain consciousness, and, over the following two or three weeks, his condition steadily deteriorated; he was put on a life-support machine and had a tracheotomy to help his breathing.

Superficially he was brain-dead. In fact, there were those who said just that, with the associated implications. After three to four weeks there was a suspicion of a twitch of an eyelid when somebody who was familiar to him made a significant comment which stimulated a 'sleeping' memory cell relating to his past. The eyelid twitch was so minimal that it did little to rekindle anything more than the slightest hope of a recovery, but it marked the turning point.

Thanks to dedicated nursing and medical skills which might well be described as being without equal, that first eyelid twitch developed into actual vision, though without any other ability to communicate for a considerable time.

Over the following two months his miraculous recovery gathered pace. At first he had little recollection of his immediate pre-operative life, though was aware of his earlier professional life. He had no recollection of his current home (where he had lived for some 10 years), showed all the classic symptoms of long-term retrograde amnesia and was totally confused as to how much time had elapsed.

Initially there was fear that his long-term memory had been virtually eliminated, like the shell of a burned-out mansion where a few parts of the structure are recognisable.

However, the most important development was that he re-learned and rebuilt his memory as a child might; fortunately, his ability to lay down 'new growth' memory had been saved. As might be expected, his short-term memory recovered first, so that he could converse with a visitor and remember his name, but was unable to recall the visit shortly afterwards.

One early and notable characteristic in his convalescence was that his intelligence appeared to be unimpaired, and, subject to the memory limitation, he was an excellent witness, describing his current and recent impressions faultlessly. He has now, after more than a year, relearned and rebuilt his ability to memorise events, as well as being able to recall most of his early memories. Today he is once more rational and, within limitations, can be analytical about much of his illness as it has been told to him, rather like reconstructing and restoring the old burned-out building.

An important contributory factor in his recovery was the character and strength of his personality, a determination, or single-mindedness, including an intriguing doggedness which had, in earlier years, made him into one of the most renowned forwards to play in the Cambridge rugby football team in the 1930s.

He still complains about his old inability to remember names, but plays bridge most competently!

Full mobility took some time to return, but much of this was probably due to his new hip which had not received the attention it would normally have received.

The likely explanation of his PVS could be that there was a temporary shutdown of a critical portion of his intra-cranial blood supply which just stopped short of a total cut-off. Such phenomena have been increasingly reported in medical journals as following major surgery and especially following heart surgery. It is often attributed to a fat embolism.

This man probably came as near to death as anybody I have met, but as far as I know, he had no illusory recollections to report from 'the other side'.

Memory obliteration can be likened to an archaeological dig: when the brain suffers damage of a non-permanent nature, (long-term) memory is removed in layers. This may be temporary or permanent.

Concussion, following a blow to the head, such as might happen in a game of football or in a fall, comes into this category. The brain is shaken up and the incident may or may not be accompanied by loss of consciousness. The victim may protest that he is all right and even wander around, but on being questioned he appears blank and has no idea where he is, why he is there, or what has been happening for some hours prior to the incident; this is called retrograde amnesia, and the sufferer needs careful treatment for twenty-four hours in case deterioration takes place, possibly due to intra-cranial bleeding.

I was taught as a medical student that no head injury is so slight that it can be ignored, nor so serious that all hope is abandoned.

Any memory impairment, however brief, is an indication for watching the victim closely for twenty-four hours.

There does not have to be a physical blow to cause the damage; a virus infection can cause even more devastating effects than a severe blow. Whatever the cause, the degree of damage to the memory may well occur in time layers. Relatively minor damage, as in concussion, merely removes, sometimes permanently, all memory of events immediately prior to the damaging incident (retrograde amnesia).

A more serious incident may remove all recollection of events, not only for a much longer time prior to the event, but also to a greater degree. For example, depending on the depth of the original impression, a victim may recall a significant event that took place earlier in his life, such as when he was a teacher or a musician or any profession which had required considerable study or experience; but he may have no recollection of a single event which happened on a single day such as having been to the theatre – he may not even recognise the theatre itself.

Brain damage may result from a wide variety of causes:

a) Trauma, as in a blow or injury to the skull.

b) Mechanical, as when a part of the brain is deprived of oxygen. This may be of a temporary nature, when full recovery may take place, or more permanent, when recovery is less likely.

c) Destruction, due to a bursting of a large blood vessel.

d) Replacement of brain tissue as in a brain tumour or other 'space-occupying lesion'.

e) Infection by a virus, when the resultant damage may vary widely.

f) Post-surgical damage, when during an operation on any part of the body (but especially likely to occur during open-heart surgery) minute fragments of tissue or blood clots or blood components (such as fat particles) may lodge in a small blood vessel.

The effects of the above causes, and the list is by no means exhaustive, vary enormously, from paralysis down the whole side of a body (usually termed a 'stroke' in lay language) through extended unconsciousness, even simulating 'clinical brain-death', to a total personality change, with possibly violent mood swings or even epilepsy.

The consequences of brain damage, according to the wider ramifications of the term are endless, but some examples from my case notes will illustrate the importance of understanding the small, but sometimes serious consequences of brain illness.

Case One

A blow to the head following a fall from a horse: the rider got to her feet at once, but could not understand why she was dressed in riding clothes, for what she recollected was that she was supposed to be at the hairdresser's prior to going out to meet an old school friend that evening. After a night in bed she was able to recall going to the stables and preparing her horse, but nothing further. Her memory of the ride itself was permanently obliterated.

Case Two

A senior underwriter at Lloyd's had a relatively minor road accident: he was unconscious for three weeks, and, on gradually regaining consciousness, he suffered from varying degrees of memory loss, although knew his family and was soon able to regain his mobility. In this case, however, his personality had changed and for several weeks he was completely unable to make the simplest of decisions, such as choosing what to have for a meal. He subsequently made a full recovery.

Case Three

A man walked into a police station, asking for assistance to find out who, and what he was. He had no identifying papers on him, and was not able to say what town he was in, or how he had got there. He thought that his name was John. He was able to carry out normal tasks 'in the moment', was fully mobile, could go to the toilet and feed himself and talk rationally, even knowing something about current affairs. He was referred to a rehabilitation centre which is where I saw him.

After three weeks rehabilitation a fair idea of what skills he was able to demonstrate emerged, but there was no clue as to his earlier background. Eventually, after some publicity, a woman claimed him as her husband, and he eventually recognised who she was. It then emerged that there had been a great emotional family crisis and it was concluded that this was a case of hysteria and he was allowed to return home.

Case Four

(This was featured on television, but I saw the patient in connection with an attendance allowance application.)

An intelligent middle-aged man with nothing untoward in his history was a senior producer in the BBC. An accomplished musician, he was in the middle of a most promising career. One day he suffered what was thought to be a slight cold, but which turned out to be a viral infection, presumably in his brain. After a few days he recovered fully, at least physically, but his short-term memory was virtually non-existent. This meant that, unlike long-term memory destruction, he knew who he was and what he was and who his family were; he had lost none of his skills, but due to his short-term memory ability being destroyed he was unable to remember appointments or days or anything recently learned or acquired. In practical terms he would be unable to find his way around out of doors or to conduct a conversation, as he would have forgotten what it was about by the end of the sentence.

Life became very frustrating and he needed constant caring for. On the occasions when his wife visited him in hospital and would leave him for a few minutes before returning to his room, he would greet her rapturously, asking, "Where have you been all this time – I haven't seen you for weeks."

On meeting him and explaining why I had come to see him, having been introduced by the ward sister, he would repeatedly ask who and what I was and why I was there.

He had just enough short-term memory to be able to find his way to the toilet – in other words, oft-repeated, straightforward routes could be re-learned. Sometimes he would confuse himself and then become irritable. He was in the habit of playing patience a great deal, and when I saw him doing this I asked if he played a lot, to which he replied that he never played cards nowadays!

If he were to go into the street, he would get hopelessly lost, and was picked up by the police.

He needed a mental 'crutch', just as a physically disabled person needs a pair of crutches. Being a skilled musician he was able to conduct an orchestra, and when asked what his work was would emphatically reply that he was a 'musical producer at the BBC', quite correct, though outdated.

Living totally in, and for the immediate present, with little or no recollection of the immediate past, he was in a time warp. Being in command of his faculties, he was therefore constantly frustrated. Try and imagine yourself in the same position. Time has effectively stopped.

It is as though you are standing on a single step of a moving staircase (the present) and you stay there: you are aware that your environment is changing, advertisements passing by, and people going in the opposite direction. By the time you reach the end of the escalator it is most unlikely that you can recall any of these passing events, such as the advertisements or people, without a special reason for doing so. For a period, you have lived in the immediate present, on that particular step you have been standing on, albeit it a moving step, though without any connection between one moment and the next.

But, as in the case of our patient, the immediate time continues, in so far as the next mealtime will come around. You will become tired so you know that it is time for bed; bodily needs issue their message so you will make an effort to recall where the toilet is and probably have no difficulty over this as it is a repetitive happening over short periods of time.

Being encapsulated in the present you will be unable to make any plans, for plans for personal forward planning are essentially built on past events, but you have no immediate past. You might attempt to keep a diary, but this would only serve to exacerbate your frustration, for none of the entries would have any meaning.

You would progressively lose contact with those you have loved, your family and friends, for, although you would recall their faces from the pre-memory loss days, friendships need revitalising from time to time and your ability to converse about current matters would have ceased. With the passage of time they would all progressively become older than your memory recalled, and, like Jonathan Swift's Luggnuggians in Laputaland, you would increasingly feel more isolated and out of touch with everything. The chances are that with increasing frustration you would tend to withdraw (does this explain the repetitive card playing?), irritable, and possibly suicidal.

This man will require a degree of care and attention for the rest of his life just as great as the 'waking coma' cases require.

Case Five

This was an example of a 'waking coma'. Such cases usually start with a blow to the head, often in a car accident, which might leave no outward evidence of any physical injury. I was called to see this particular young man several months after his injury. He lived with his parents in a deserted farmhouse just outside Swindon.

When I saw him, his parents had set up a very caring routine and made a special 'day bed' with every form of equipment for turning him, and devices ('ripple bed') to prevent pressure sores. There was no sign of consciousness, although he would respond to a hard pinch, in which case that limb would be withdrawn. His eyes were sometimes open but without any evidence of sight. His mother said that just occasionally she might discern some recognition when she spoke to him by name, when his eyelids might make a slight movement.

Otherwise he would not make any movement and had to be fed through a tube. To establish a routine, his parents would turn him every half hour, and transfer him to another ('night') bed at the appropriate time. There was an impression that bodily 'night' was different to 'day'. He was doubly incontinent.

I was told that he was an only child and had lived all his life with his parents. He had had no particularly dangerous habits but helped his parents on an isolated farm and was interested in motor cars. One night after the family had retired to bed the telephone had rung, and he had been heard to get out of bed and go the garage and drive off in the family car.

Early the next morning the postman had arrived with the police to tell them that their car had hit a tree with some resultant damage, and that their son had been found in the driving seat without any evident external injuries, although he was unconscious, from which state he had never recovered.

The wider effect on the family of this not uncommon story has to be seen to be understood. I saw this man once more about a year later, before hearing that he had died of a chest infection some three years after his accident.

'Waking Coma' Cases

Invariably these cases are caused by physical injuries in one form or another; these are usually road traffic accidents but may occur in other arenas such as hunting or in any potentially violent sports. Though unconscious, the victims may have little or no visible sign of an injury.

The prognosis of these waking coma cases is uncertain and causes great distress to the families. The damage is usually to the brainstem and often due to varying degrees of brain haemorrhage. Treatment, apart from intensive physical care, is to attempt to 'arouse' the 'sleeping' brain by different forms of stimuli. A reason for this is that, whilst in this state, the patient lacks any form of stimulus from the special senses, i.e., hearing or sight or smell, from the outside world. It is as though they are cocooned, and treatment aims at breaking through the 'envelope ' in which the patient is engulfed. One way is to hold the patient tightly and speak familiar and welcoming sounds, not dissimilar to the technique one might use when trying to rouse somebody from a very deep sleep. Indeed a 'waking coma' can be regarded as an extreme version of deep sleep.

The chances of recovery diminish after six months, and if no progress has taken place after twelve months the case can be regarded as hopeless.

This is an area causing the greatest heart-searching when the ultimate disposal is considered. Legal history was made in the case of Tony Bland who was pronounced brain-dead following the Hillsborough football disaster, when he was crushed against a fence, depriving his brain of vital oxygen. In due course, the courts ruled that it would be justifiable to turn off his feeding tubes, leaving his body to die after a few weeks. Surely a more humane and cleaner way must be found to give such cases a more dignified ending?

Legal history has been made so progress must inevitably follow.

Chapter Sixteen
Brain Failure – Alzheimer's Disease

This is such a common disease and it is increasing as the number of old people increases, so it needs special attention. It is the common cause of senile dementia, is more common in females, and rarely seen before the age of 45. When the symptoms develop before the age of 60 it is called pre-senile dementia.

It is rare for those afflicted with the illness to know what is wrong with themselves, because, by the time the illness is established sufficiently to be noticed by relatives, the ability for self-assessment has gone. Prior to this point being reached, the victim has developed techniques of deception and plausibility to a degree which deceives all but the most discerning observer.

Of nearly 700 cases of Alzheimer's that came across my own path I can recall only two cases where the sufferer had the remotest idea of what was afoot, perhaps because they were both medically qualified.

One, a retired GP, probably had a hunch at an early stage in his illness. One morning he shouted to his wife that he was unable to tie his tie however hard he tried. 'I get in a muddle when I attempt to thread the end through the loop.' Apart from his poor memory, which he put down to lack of mental exercise and a disinclination to meet people, he led a simple, if quiet life, listening to music, which, perhaps significantly, caused him to sleep a lot during the day.

"Perhaps I'm getting senile dementia!" he joked, though one wonders how serious he was, and, together with his arthritic wife, he became a resident in a residential home some months later, where I saw him as a rather forgetful and inactive man.

The other case, also medically qualified, had reason to hide his fears, for he worked part-time in the California State Highways Department on road safety, although everybody seemed to have forgotten about his existence in a small back office. When eventually he was 'rustled out' on account of his strange timekeeping and because of a near miss whilst driving, he was clearly not well enough to continue in his 'research' task.

On clearing up his desk, a scrap of paper was discovered in his desk drawer, with row upon row of a nearly indecipherable single word written upon it: it was the word 'Alzheimer's' written line after line.

A characteristic failing is an inability to interpret angles. As angles are fundamental to many visual skills this is most significant, placing the victim at a great disadvantage. A clock face cannot be read because of the angles at which the clock hands are, giving the first message of 'time'. The victim ceases to wind up his watch, but continues to wear it as an ornament, so a stopped watch may be revealing to the diagnosis.

Similarly, many letters of the alphabet form angles (A, B, E, F, K, etc.), and so reading becomes incomprehensible. As a defence in trying to keep up appearances the victim will continue to look at a paper or book, but it may be the wrong way up, or the page never turned.

Alzheimer's disease is a lonely illness. The victims feel deserted, as though they live in a cocoon, with fears that they are being left to their own fate. Within their own world, fears are harboured, and, with some justification, they feel that they are unable to keep up with things.

Perhaps one way of trying to understand how they feel would be for them to write a diary of their thoughts over a period of many months but, unfortunately, they would not be able to write!

In nearly every case, one of the earliest symptoms is that the memory noticeably starts to fail. As this is a 'normal' characteristic of advancing years, it would not in itself give cause for concern, and so, coupled with the early characteristic of poor self-assessment, it would be dismissed and even laughed about in the early stages.

Entries from the imaginary diaries of Alzheimer's victims might well be written over a period of two to three years in the following terms:

1) *It is extraordinary how difficult it is to remember people's names nowadays, but the main thing is that everybody else seems to remember mine. Old 'what's-*

her-name' was pretty rude, accusing me of not seeing her the other day in the High Street. I don't recall going into the High Street anyway.

2) *People are intolerant about my handwriting, which was never very good anyway, but now I have arthritis I suppose it's not terribly good, indeed, I missed an appointment because I couldn't read my diary.*

3) *I keep losing things I have just picked up and forget why I wanted them.*

4) *I find leaving something on the stairs most helpful but cannot always remember why I left it there.*

5) *I do wish things would not keep changing, such as telephone numbers and postcodes (never could understand these anyway). I like a good rigid routine, it makes for a tidy life.*

6) *Tried to help with the housework today but I can't understand why my daughter stopped me using the Hoover on the front lawn.*

7) *Caught sight of myself in a shop window, didn't recognise myself, but I just know I look 25 years younger than that old woman.*

8) *A bit of fun this afternoon: nice-looking girl on the bus; I rather fancied her but she didn't respond to my hand. Well perhaps I should have gone a bit more gently, ah well, you can't win 'em all; but there was no need for the police constable to come round to the house, and then he called me 'granddad', all very inappropriate.*

9) *I dialled 999 yesterday, for a car stopped right outside my house and I felt sure the driver was going to break a window. The police said all he was doing was waiting for the lights to change.*

10) *I hate throwing things away: during the war we simply kept everything. My son didn't approve of my not flushing the loo (to save water) and after a week of this he was quite shirty!*

11) *Was embarrassed about a week later, was 'caught short' and, as I couldn't find the loo, did it in a flower pot, but forgot about it. I overheard my son-in-law talking about a divorce if I didn't leave; I don't want a divorce, as my old man has been good to me and I can't understand when my daughter tells me that he died many years ago; I swear I saw him only the other day.*

12) *My daughter has got a lot older. When I called her 'Mother' the other day, she seemed quite upset.*

13) *Reading is difficult; I can't remember what went on a few sentences back. My son asked why I was reading the book 'upside down'! I told him I would read the book any way that I liked, but he didn't seem to understand. Not that it matters very much as I seem to fall asleep easily in the day.*

14) *Nights have become more difficult and I don't sleep very well, but the thoughtful BBC night programmes are good. The other night my son-in-law came into my room to complain at the noise and I couldn't think why he had pyjamas on for a moment.*

15) *These long winter nights are difficult; the other night I got dressed (well, more or less) and let myself out to go to the shops. However they were all closed, and there were not many people about, which I found strange. A police car picked me up (they seem to know me quite well nowadays) and took me home. Apparently I had forgotten to put a skirt on or something.*

16) *Have trouble putting my lipstick on straight, so I have given it up. In fact, it's so much easier to give up a lot of things, like brushing my hair, after all there's no law about that sort of thing and now that I'm asleep most of the day it doesn't really matter.*

17) *A strange man came to see me the other day. He can't have been to a very good school as he wanted to know who was Prime Minister, silly man – he seemed quite*

*surprised when I was able to tell him that it was
Churchill.*

18) *Being short of cupboard space I have discovered that I
can put milk in the oven, but my son-in-law seemed
upset when it boiled over and made a mess. I retorted
that he should have looked in the oven first before
switching it on. I ask you; who was right?*

19) *Depressed nowadays; I feel drained and very alone and
want to retreat into myself as people don't talk to me
much. I can't understand why I'm helped to the
lavatory. In my own mind I feel so capable and able to
run for a bus, not that I would bother to as I remember
being told 'Never run after a bus,' or... what was the
other thing now? Anyway, the bus wouldn't be going
where I wanted it to go, so I'll stay here.*

20) *Am told I'm going away 'for a holiday'. I don't feel
that it matters any more as I'm just tired of life and
don't seem to recognise anyone or anything.*

21) *It doesn't matter any more now, I think I just want it
all to end. I feel tired and just want to sleep.*

Summary:

*As I realise that I am getting older in spite of fantasies
about being young, and therefore am still able to do all
those things I enjoyed so much when I was young, the
one thing I do notice is that my sleep pattern has
altered.*

*It has altered in two predominating ways. I
remember that a typical day commenced with waking
up refreshed, and eagerly, indeed energetically, going
right through the day. It was as though the previous
night was akin to winding up a clock. Then, as
evening came around, things would slow down, and I
would be content to relax before feeling ready to go to
bed to fall asleep, until the next day started and the
cycle commenced once more.*

Now this cycle has altered, it is not so clear cut, and even reversed. Nights seem like the active part of my day. Although I will begin by falling asleep this state does not last long, as though I had reverted to the animal kingdom, and a few hours is all that is required before I wake up and feel compelled to get up and even to get dressed.

Then the daytime also is different. When sitting down, of which I find I do a great deal, I find myself drifting into a half-dream-world, not fully asleep, but my mind wanders and I imagine things which are not really happening, though I might talk, and nobody would know what I was yakking about, although at the time it seems perfectly clear to me. In this twilight sleep I wander in and out of my dream-world, bringing accounts of happenings into the waking world. I've heard people say to one another 'Of course she rambles a lot', but then, I know that, don't I? And I just smile to myself.

Post Script On Memory

It should not be forgotten that forgetfulness is a normal physiological happening, *vide* the schoolboy who forgets to take a pencil to school.

With advancing years, such lapses tend to become more frequent, even habit-forming and more complex, such as missing appointments, and forgetting names. Such manifestations, though irritating and potentially embarrassing, should still be regarded as physiological in the context of the normal ageing process. It might be likened to 'mental arthritis', making for impaired mental agility.

Far more serious is when memory impairment reaches the stage when one cannot recall the event of having done something, such as making a speech, meeting somebody, visiting the theatre.

The former might be termed commission memory failure, the latter omission memory failure.

Chapter Seventeen
The Golden Years

This chapter is called 'The Golden Years' for, as anyone who has worked with or cared for elderly persons knows, there is an abundance of kindness, wisdom and happiness to be found amongst people who are able to enjoy their retirement. It might be likened to the glow of a fire at the end of the day when the flames have died away and the warm glow of the embers are peaceful and warmth-giving. So it is with people when the heat of the bodily chemistry has gone, leaving the soul devoid of stressful challenges from the busy, competitive, bustling and overcrowded world.

Interspersed in the tranquillity and contentment there are still not-inconsiderable difficulties, as at every phase of life for that matter, so that, although many older people say that they are having the best years of their lives, the other side of the coin must also be acknowledged when living habits have to be modified to accommodate the problems associated with the older 'age'.

'Sell-By Date'

This marketing term is increasingly creeping into the English language, especially with reference to older people. This is a travesty, and does no credit to older people. Consider the facts: the phrase has been coined to meet certain legal requirements, usually in regard to food, and is welcomed by accountants especially, whose sole objective is to increase the rate of turnover of goods.

Nor does the phrase suggest, in terms of food, that it is past its best. On the contrary, many perishable items, such as meat and cheese for example (and the better wines are even more apposite), come to maturity after some time, usually after this 'date'. Whatever other connotation might be intended, it is certainly not 'unfit for human consumption' or 'useless' and so with the older human, as has been pointed out elsewhere, for, as in the sell-by date label, there are considerable advantages in acquiring such goods, as the keen shopper is aware, and these very goods are much sought after, for they offer better value. Take heed, you who are of pensionable age, you are a better bargain!

Do not assume that because someone is getting older that they have necessarily become less active. A cautionary tale: I recall a terrible *faux pas* I made and was soundly put in my place, not for the first time, by my cousin Peg, a formidable but kindly lady by any standards. On this particular day I greeted her by way of enquiring how she was (she was then in her middle 70s) and by asking if she was still playing tennis?

"Still...!" she proclaimed, in the manner of Dame Edith Evans pronouncing on the 'The Handbag' in *The Importance of Being Earnest*. This was accompanied by a withering look that would have done credit to any hypnotist wishing to see if I was worthy of further attention. Even the dog looked uneasy and asked to leave the room, so that I was left in no doubt that an apology, much less an explanation, would serve little purpose other than to entomb me.

In another section, I have discussed a selection from some 10,000 patients who were seen over some twenty years, all of whom were disabled by illness in some form or another. Some of these illnesses and accompanying disabilities are more common in older people (arthritis), but some can occur at any age (multiple sclerosis). The common denominator is disablement in some form, and some examples have been selected.

I have noticed another common denominator amongst older people – notwithstanding a variety of 'infirmities' (not all of which are obvious, as the following story illustrates), and that is a sense of humour. One elderly man – outwardly nothing wrong with him – told me that he had seen a signpost in Sussex, reading:

FOR THE CONTINENT – STRAIGHT ON VIA NEWHAVEN

Under this, some wag had added:

For the incontinent, turn right for Brighton,
and Beth's Home for the Elderly.

He recounted the story with such vigour that he shook with enjoyment, before excusing himself! It was not difficult to see that he could laugh at himself!

Physical Disabilities

Nature would appear to compensate those less fortunate who are handicapped in some way. It is as though, unable to be tempted by such things as playing games or other mobile pursuits, they concentrate their energies into other channels such as the achievement of academic excellence, the arts, or even the mastery of some form of technology.

Spina Bifida

This is a condition where the base of the spinal column is imperfectly formed, leaving the youngster (for it is present from birth) with varying degrees of paralysis from the waist down. One such teenager, confined to a wheelchair, succeeded in persuading his friends that it was they who were disadvantaged by having so many diversionary interests, tempting them much as a puppy will be drawn to chewing a slipper or (as he put it) even a live electric cable, with the attendant risks. It was this same boy who scoffed at the idea of having separate sections in the Olympics for 'disabled' people: 'If I want to compete with anyone, it will be on my terms at my own speciality, and I will make sure I win.'

Cerebral Palsy

This is a condition which, although the intellect is unimpaired, causes severe speech defects, almost to the point of unintelligibility and is accompanied with difficulty in moving limbs in a precise manner, thus putting severe stress on the afflicted person, aggravated by the way people assume (s)he is incapable of rational thought, a typical example of 'Does he take sugar?' syndrome.

One such case I visited in his home had turned himself into a recluse, but when I entered his attic home I discovered the nature of his reclusive lifestyle.

He was confined to a wheelchair and relied upon kindly neighbours to bring him the essentials of life. He had turned his single room into a communication Aladdin's cave, filled with sophisticated ham radio equipment, and spent several hours each day communicating with every country in the world. Paradoxically his speech impediment was not in evidence when he was talking 'blind' to fellow hams. He claimed to know over 100 fellow enthusiasts around the world, including one head of state. Living his life in semi-darkness, surrounded by his high-tech radio and other advanced electronic equipment was made possible by tapping into a wide variety of grants from central as well as local government. He was a burden to nobody; the world was at the command of his ears and fingers; his body became a mere 'residence' from which he could communicate with his friends at all times of the day or night.

As a listening post he was able on more than one occasion to render a service to his fellow beings by picking up mayday calls on his radio, and had even been in touch with astronauts in space. His disability was of little consequence to him, indeed he considered that without it his life would have been the poorer.

Speech Impediment

Try and imagine that you want to know the way to a station. You stop a lady in the street, and start, "Gggggggggg. Gggggg. Gggg" You pause and, making a valiant effort, start again "Gggan yyyyyyyyou pppppppppp..." You give up and walk away, having attracted a small hostile crowd.

What would your chances of employment be?

One such patient was a youngster; just after he had left school, he was determinedly trying to get employment, but without success because his very severe stammer made him unemployable. I was asked to make some suggestions; ironically, the cure was related to noise, the louder the better.

He had succeeded at school, for, as he put it, you learn by watching and listening and pass exams by writing; finding employment was more difficult as an ability to talk suddenly became all important. I first came across him, or, to be exact, became aware of his existence, when he elected to phone me at home, which was a total failure. He was in a phone box and I heard the sound of money being inserted, and then all I could hear was a succession of splutterings; no speech, but occasionally the splutterings would cease, to be replaced by the sound of more cash being inserted, and then more incoherent noises until even they ceased.

I reported my phone as being out of order, and thought little more about it until I received a letter from this young man asking for an appointment. His name was John, and at that time I was doing a number of medical examinations for industrial rehabilitation.

John turned out to be a most amiable youngster although not by his conversation, which was virtually non-existent. He resorted to writing everything down, but his personality was 'alive' and I agreed to try and help him. As, several consultations later, I managed to establish a sort of rapport with him, finishing his sentences off for him, after the fashion of the Two Ronnies, I asked him to try and phone me at a certain time. To my astonishment (although there was a lot of background noise) he talked without hesitation, explaining that he couldn't hear *me* very well as there was a pneumatic drill in the background.

We had by chance hit upon the cure, and I recalled some work being carried out at Edinburgh University which entailed the victim wearing headsets playing back an amplification of his own voice, which had the psychological, but paradoxical effect of drowning his own speech. This worked on John, and over the next few months his self-confidence increased to the point at which he was able to talk normally without help from the 'Edinburgh box'.

Colour Blind

Accidents can be caused in most unexpected ways.

I was asked by a construction company to advise on a recently employed youngster who had just left school a few weeks previously and whose employers were querying his mental ability. I enquired as to the nature of his work, and was told he was a labourer working on the by-pass that was being constructed nearby. I visited the site and found this youngster had been directing traffic with two flags, one red, the other green. I hurried to see him, to find that he had thrown the red flag away and couldn't understand why he had been given two flags of an identical colour with which to direct the traffic! Fortunately, such was his personality that he stopped cars by 'threatening' them with his flag, irrespective of its colour!

Brain Injuries

It would not be feasible in a book such as this to list all the possible brain or mental afflictions that might befall one with the passing of the years. Instead, I would like to show that mental 'crutches' can be as effective as physical crutches in their own way.

Angus was such an example. I was asked to evaluate him for employment after a prolonged period of treatment and rehabilitation.

His history was that, some years previously, he had been operating a circular saw, cutting up wood. A large length of wood had become detached, and, like a spear, had penetrated up through the roof of his mouth and into his brain, causing a terrible wound, but miraculously not killing him, although he had been unconscious for some time. He also lost two fingers on his right hand.

Miraculously, Angus recovered, although with two residual handicaps. He had undergone a personality change, becoming moody and irritable, perhaps not surprisingly. Another, and more significant change was a severe memory defect; he could no longer remember numbers and names, which is a characteristic all too often found in the elderly (and sometimes not so elderly) in lesser degrees. His ability to reason was unimpaired and he used this to good advantage in overcoming his memory failure as the following experiment demonstrated when I was asked to assess him at a rehabilitation centre.

He was briefly shown a card with the figures '854' written on it and asked to memorise it. Some time later he was asked to repeat the number. Angus gazed into the distance as though seeking inspiration, counting his fingers, and his lips moving without uttering a sound, as though he was reasoning something out. After about a minute his eyes lit up with satisfaction and he said, "854."

I was astonished and enquired how he did it.

He explained that it was perfectly simple. He knew his memory was poor (it was virtually non-existent), so that, when faced with a challenge, he would devise a mental 'prop' around which he could proceed step by step, which, in this matter, proceeded thus:

i)   I only have three fingers on my right hand, that reminds me that the number has three digits.

ii) I was born on the 17th day of a month: $1+7=8$, i.e., the first number.

iii) Subtract 8 from $17 = 9$.

iv) 9 is the sum of the last two digits, so divide by 2, which in rational order gives 5 and $4 = 854$.

Angus illustrates how somebody with a specific disability, rather than general debility, is able to show resourcefulness in overcoming his handicap.

Blind or Deaf – Which?

One often ponders which might be the more disabling: total blindness or total deafness. In the course of my career I had the opportunity to find out, as I saw several hundred cases of both. Here are my conclusions.

Vision

The primary services rendered by vision are:
- i) Defensive: To warn of dangers such as 'predators' in the form of animals or insects.
- ii) Obstacle avoidance.
- iii) To provide information such as time, serving of food, and reading.
- iv) Orientation: To locate objects; to find one's way around.
- v) Appreciation: of beauty and form.
- vi) Warning: of anger or similar threats.

Hearing

The primary services rendered by sound are.
- i) Information.
- ii) Communication.
- iii) Warnings.
- iv) Retaining contact.
- v) Appreciation of art (auditory, e.g., music).

The most important of the above is:

Communication

This is essential in order to keep in contact with the world and one's fellow beings. Although hearing and vision complement and reinforce the other, hearing is the more effective of the two if only one is functioning.

Sight and hearing might be considered to be 'master senses', and not only does one reinforce the other but other special senses also, such as smell or touch and even taste (as when food 'looks good').

In the event of either of the two 'master senses' being lost, substitutes can be called into play to varying degrees; in the case of blindness especially, the sense of extrasensory perception (ESP) can sometimes be partially recovered.

'Artificial' substitutes have an important role to play: for blind people, guide dogs or a white stick, and audible warnings on pedestrian crossings. Talking books help to substitute hearing for sight and fellow beings. Strangers are not inhibited from assisting blind persons, in the same way as they might be inhibited from helping disabled persons who can see. This is probably because they (the helpers) do not feel under examination by the person in need of assistance.

In the case of deafness a feeling of isolation is common as two-way communication is severely restricted; this is partially ameliorated by utilising lip-reading, which is only possible under certain circumstances.

Coping with Blindness

In a hostile or unfriendly environment sight plays a much more critical role than in a civilised community. Examples of auditory warnings in a developed country have been cited: auditory warnings on pedestrian crossings, and bells or electronic beepers on public transport, indicating doors which are about to close. Blind people can name many more examples of how sound helps them to avoid dangers, and interpret changes taking place around them which will enable them to orientate themselves. Familiarity with the surroundings plays an important part in orientation.

For the blind person, hands and fingers can play a part in passing information to the brain, via switches for example, and even cooking can be done. A sightless person becomes more tactile and uses his fingers in the manner of an insect using antennae.

There will be shortcomings, but even some of these can be overcome. There will be no awareness of colour matching, but clothes can be segmented in specific drawers so that differently coloured garments can be selected.

Warnings and 'attention getters' can be transmitted aurally, and the doorbell or telephone bell retain their customary functions.

Most importantly, information is easier to assimilate by sound than by visual means, so communication with the world is relatively unimpaired, with a little adaptation.

Now try to consider the plight of someone who is totally deaf by trying a simple experiment on yourself.

Switch on your television set, almost any type of programme will do; now cover the picture up and measure the time that it takes to pick up and follow the thread of the programme. Next, reverse the process, and switch off the sound. Convinced?

In both blindness and deafness the age at which the person loses the facility affects how (s)he will be able to adapt. If either blindness or deafness is congenital, then the disability is as minimal as it can be, in the sense that what you have never had you have never missed, and alternative compensatory 'senses' can be developed with any available communication channels. Lost vision can be compensated for far more easily than can lost hearing, and by less drastic means, as illustrated by the following story.

Congenital deafness and therefore hearing having never been experienced, may be brought about by the mother catching German measles at a critical stage in pregnancy, causing the infant to be born completely deaf. Learning to speak is nearly impossible, for hearing one's own speech plays an important part in the initial stages of learning to speak, and so a critical communication in the learning phase of life is missing.

I met such a congenitally deaf four-year-old child in Swindon, who was oblivious to traffic, as she could not hear the traffic sounds. Being of normal intelligence she became aware at an early age that traffic should be associated with danger, but she was also aware that people listened for approaching traffic – a facility which she did not have. To her mother's horror she found her daughter placing her ear to the ground so that she might detect the vibrations of an approaching vehicle!

Coping with Deafness

A deaf person is virtually isolated. Their attention is more difficult to catch unless they happen to be looking at the attention-seeking source. Two-way communication is more difficult to start and to maintain.

'Auditory' arts are more flexible and more lasting than visual arts. The visual sense soon dulls and can only be perceived for a relatively short (finite) period, except for mobile events (such as sporting events), in which case a spoken commentary can serve as a substitute.

Music, being variable, can be appreciated for longer periods than visual objects.

My own conclusion was decided by a 70-year-old totally blind man who lived in Northleach in Gloucestershire, whom I first met as a patient in his home. He could invariably be seen standing on the pavement in the centre of Northleach 'watching' the world go by, with his guide dog sitting patiently by his side. He would greet all passers-by by their names, and to my astonishment when I walked past, he said, "Good Morning, Doctor," although I had not seen him for nearly a year!

I stopped to pass the time of day, asking what he had been doing. His reply was revealing. He mentioned a number of persons by name whom he had 'seen' that morning.

He was not 'blind' (except in the technical meaning of the word), since he was in close touch with the world!

In contrast, deaf people resort to dominating the conversation because they are unable to listen and they retain the initiative, doing all the talking! And to show that deafness is not the handicap that might be supposed, I well recall a strong but delightful lady (one Dame Kathleen Ollerenshaw) for whom I have the highest respect, who, if the conversation was not going to her liking, would abruptly switch off her hearing-aid and then guide the subject to her satisfaction! But then she still had her hearing whenever she needed it, and she knew its value!

Skill Fatigue

This is a manifestation peculiar to the older person. It might be called the 'absent-minded professor syndrome'.

As the years accumulate so the ability to do several tasks simultaneously diminishes, and undivided attention to a single task is needed if the thread of the task is not to be lost. Women retain this 'multiple task' ability much longer and more effectively than men.

Perhaps the condition is epitomised by the apocryphal story concerning GK Chesterton, when he left home to deliver a most important lecture. Several hours later, to his wife's dismay, though not surprise, she received a telegram: 'Am at Crewe. Where should I be?'

The question often comes up as to whether an elderly individual should still be driving. Sometimes the matter is brought to a head through a minor accident and the offender is ordered to retake a driving test.

What is happening in such cases is quite simple. Even at a relatively early stage in life, such a state can happen to anybody, but especially if the same route is frequently followed. Should a minor deviation be needed, to go via a certain shop for example, the journey is commenced and the driving skill is relegated to 'autopilot'; it is only at some later stage that the driver realises that he is on a different road to that required.

So with an elderly driver. This person may be driving along and stops at a red traffic light, meanwhile thinking about something totally irrelevant to the task in hand. His dream is rudely shattered by the driver behind sounding his horn aggressively and on looking up he sees the lights at green, but by the time he gets the car into gear, in his agitation possibly stalling the engine, and restarts it again he blunders off at full power, quite oblivious of the fact the lights have turned to red again.

Chapter Eighteen
Exitus or Voluntary Euthanasia

Definition: *'The bringing about of a gentle and easy death in the case of incurable and painful disease'.*

Lord let me know my end, and what is the measure of my days:
Let me know how fleeting my life is and realise my frailty'.

Psalm 39 v. 5.

No treatise covering the subject of how long one might, and more relevantly, could, or even should live would be complete without touching, however briefly, upon the topic of voluntary euthanasia.

Though it is perfectly proper, indeed important, to touch on the subject, I believe it would be impertinent to make any recommendations or even pronouncements about the morality of voluntary euthanasia, for of all the decisions one makes during life this is the most personal and critical of them all, and is literally the last decision one can make before the end.

During the course of life most people think about living and how to improve one's lot, material or otherwise, and perhaps how to improve someone else's lot, and they generally look forward to and plan the future.

The principal consideration one gives to death is how to defer it, although even this must sometimes be questioned, given how some people behave in their lifestyles, especially on the roads.

As the journey through life progresses, the emphasis gradually and almost imperceptibly shifts from the longer term future to the more immediate future, including the possibility of death, then to the probability, and eventually to the inevitability of death.

So a brief reference to voluntary euthanasia has a place here, leaving the ultimate decision, where feasible, to each individual.

There came a point in my life, as doubtless it has to many others, when I was beginning to philosophise occasionally, not consciously, but indirectly, about the different exit routes, and wondering what the Grim Reaper had in store for me. Doubtless this was helped by seeing so many of my patients near to life's journey's end and discussing it with them, in many cases quite freely. It was striking to find that at this stage few were frightened at the thought of dying, but rather the method and 'quality' of dying.

Then, one day, I chanced on meeting Jean Davies, at that time the honorary secretary of the Voluntary Euthanasia Society (VES)[1], and was impressed by her rational, even cheerful approach to the whole subject. As the result, I became a life member of the VES, and found myself amongst a very jolly, down-to-earth body of people.

I felt unable to accept the invitation to join their committee at the time as I felt it was incompatible with the appointment I then held as Head of the St John Ambulance, as the one's primary concern was how to save life and the other's how to terminate it.

Having joined the VES – as a life member! – I then resumed the enjoyment of living and, surprisingly, and more significantly, worried much less about my own death, once I had arranged for my 'advance declaration', or 'living will' to be completed.

History of Euthanasia

An extract from an article in the VES newsletter by a group of students (Claire Alo et al.) at the University of Brighton: I am grateful to Ms Shui-Fong NG for permission to reproduce.

> *Socrates saw painful disease and suffering as a good reason not to cling to life. In Rome, ending one's life because of terminal illness was considered a good act. Seneca, the Stoic, wrote: 'It makes a great deal of difference whether a man is lengthening his life or his*

---

[1] The Voluntary Euthanasia Society, 13 Prince of Wales Terrace, London W8 5PG, Tel: 0171 376 2648.

death. But if the body is useless for service, why should not one free a struggling soul?'

But in the second and third centuries, developments in Christian thinking went the other way, and St Thomas Aquinas wrote of euthanasia as the most dangerous of sins, in violation of the Sixth Commandment, as well as leaving no time for repentance, and thus it remained for twelve centuries.

In 1516, Sir Thomas More's Utopia *depicted a world in which voluntary euthanasia was officially sanctioned. Meanwhile, advances in medicine meant patients could be kept alive for longer, but at the price of increased suffering.*

In the early nineteenth century Karl Marx criticised physicians who treated the disease and not the patient when they could not find a cure.

Acceptance of voluntary euthanasia received a setback in the first part of the 20th century when the Nazis murdered thousands of mentally and physically handicapped Germans under the label of 'euthanasia', and it is only recently that there have been moves to make voluntary euthanasia more acceptable in the Western world, with special reference to Holland.

The mood for and against voluntary euthanasia has swung to and fro, but there are now signs that it is becoming more acceptable as legislation is gradually being introduced throughout the world. A major step forward occurred when, in Britain, legislation was passed making it illegal to countermand a patient's wish not to be given treatment, and, if this is disregarded, then an assault is deemed to have been committed.

I believe that a fillip would be given to the movement if the society were to resume the use of their former name – EXIT – which puts matters quite sharply and succinctly, rather than VES.

As at present drawn up, the 'law is an ass' state of affairs exists. Take two identical patients, both suffering from incurable painful and intolerable illness.

Both have requested that they be allowed, even helped to die, and there is no question about their sincerity, and no lack of understanding about their wishes.

The respective physicians both respect their patients' wishes, and want to help. One gives increasing doses of a painkilling drug, and in due course the patient (call him Brown), dies.

Everybody is satisfied that the right thing has been done.

The doctor to the other patient (Smith) achieves the same end by injecting insulin, which is not a painkiller, nor for that matter is it a help for any condition from which Smith is suffering. It does, however, terminate Smith's life, indeed very quickly, and you might say it was preferable to that which happened to Brown who lived for several days, albeit in a coma, thus prolonging the family's distress.

The result was that both patients were released from intolerable suffering in accord with their wishes. The families were relieved and released from their anxiety for their relative, even though neither knew, nor did they wish to know, the precise details of treatment.

However, the coroner was informed and the police started making enquiries and, following a post-mortem, it was discovered that Smith had been 'killed' by an overdose of insulin, and the physician was charged with a criminal act.

For myself, I have made my wishes to my physician perfectly clear; I have discussed it with my GP and my family, and we all well know what to do (if necessary) when the time comes.

I will conclude by repeating: I make no recommendations except to decide what your own views and wishes may be, and, for those who so choose, a specimen 'advance declaration' is reproduced.

TO MY FAMILY AND MY PHYSICIAN

This declaration is made by me, ...

....

at a time when I am of sound mind and after careful consideration.

If the time comes when I can no longer take part in decisions for my own future, let this declaration stand as the testament to my wishes:

If there is no reasonable prospect of my recovery from physical illness or impairment expected to cause me severe distress OR to render me incapable of rational existence, I request that I be allowed to die and not be kept alive by artificial means and that I receive whatever quantity of drugs may be required to keep me free from pain or distress even if the moment of death is hastened.

This declaration is signed and dated by me in the presence of the two under-mentioned witnesses present at the same time who, at my request, in my presence and in the presence of each other, have hereto subscribed their names as witnesses.

Signed ....
Date ....

First Witness's Signature..
Name ....
Address ....
....
Occupation ....

Second Witness's Signature..
Name ....
Address ....
....
Occupation ....

NOTE: Witnesses should not be members of the family.

Epilogue

*A lifetime of happiness: No man could bear it:
It would be Hell on Earth.*

George Bernard Shaw.

Having heard the views of over ten thousand patients, whilst I have prodded them, listened to them, shared sorrows with them and invariably respected them, I return to the question:

Why not live a little longer?

Any answer will depend upon so many different and varying factors, such as age, the state of health, the quality of life, the social circumstances, and the personality varying from day to day with mood swings.

We will now see whether it is possible to answer the question, 'Why not live a little longer?'

I admit that I have doubts about there being a definitive answer!

If you have managed to 'stay the course' by reading the whole of this book, you will be aware that the text has led you through a wide variety of scenes, many of which may remind you of similar experiences in your own life, for nobody's life is wholly unique, even though it might vary in detail.

One thing is certain: the objective of living a little longer should not solely be the pursuit of eternal and perpetual happiness, as Bernard Shaw aptly put it.

Life is an amalgam of all sorts of experiences, some happy, some sad, a little pain mixed with some pleasure, the sum total of which makes for life's rich pageantry.

Perhaps that is as near as one can get to finding an answer to the question. When the richness of the pageantry begins to fade beyond recognition, then and only then and not before should one contemplate the question in the negative.

A Visit to the Dentist and Immortality

How long *would* you like to live for? Would you like to live for ever? Some people light-heartedly say it would be fun, and interesting to watch how the world might develop. Fun?

To find an answer, I would ask you to join me in my dentist's chair. I must explain that I am fortunate in having the best dentist in London. For professional reasons he would not permit me to give his professional name and address, but as he is also a very dear friend, I can tell you that the name of my friend is Keith Kemp. Should you deduce the name of my dentist from this, I commend you, as – for the moment at least – I can assure you that you do not appear to be suffering from advanced cerebral disease. However, do not assume that more sophisticated tests would reach the same reassuring conclusion. (By the way, do you recall the name of that fellow you met last week? No? But how about the initials of somebody in your class at school? Yes? Surprised? Don't worry, I expect you know your present telephone number – you can always call for help should your memory deteriorate much further!)

As to my dentist's address, well... I'm quite unable to tell you precisely, as I don't know Lower Sloane Street very well, but he was always grumbling about how like 'pieces of *eight*' the inside of my mouth was.

As I settled into the dentist's chair (it reminded me of those electric chairs used for executions), and as the dental nurse tied a 'bib' around my neck, I was reflecting on how dental records are frequently consulted as an aid to the identification of a corpse, no matter how long the owner has been dead. It was as though a dentist carried out their repair work with such diligence that it was intended to last forever; as indeed it did, though not necessarily remaining functional. In this sense, a dentist's work is unique in the field of medicine, though ironically it doesn't carry a lifetime guarantee. Curious, as Alice might have mused.

My dentist has the happy knack of being quite unflappable, and everybody I have met appears delighted to visit him. I once asked him what might be the secret of his popularity, knowing that a visit to the dentist was usually viewed with a mixture of dread and horror.

"Oh, it's really quite simple," he said. "I've indoctrinated all my patients to view a visit to the doctor as being something to dread much more than coming here, as they can be pretty sure that I will only be examining one orifice, whereas a doctor... well, have you ever worked out how many orifices a doctor has to choose from..." His voice trailed away, as he invited me to "Open a little wider please..."

Peering in an exploratory way into my mouth in the manner of a small boy prodding amongst the rock pools at low tide (I have often been tempted to hide a small treasure amongst my teeth for him to find), I heard him mutter, "These should see him out," and he continued polishing with what I can only describe as something akin to being exposed to Concorde's Olympus engines with reheat fully alight. At the command, "Rinse." I asked him how long he had designed his examination-cum-repair work to last for. His reply was succinct. "Long after your interest in mastication has gone, and I would refer you to Jonathan Swift."

On the further command, "Rinse please," I estimated that I had approximately nine seconds in which to phrase a question – if I gurgled my speech and couched it in 'telegram language' – before being 'laid to rest' once more in the supine position, accompanied by a dying gurgle. As I once more gazed at my dentist's masked face a few inches away from my mouth, closing my eyes (does everybody close their eyes at this juncture?), I pondered whether my dentist ever imagined he was giving the last rites? I tried to think of more pleasant happenings as the drill created a kaleidoscope of colour before my tightly closed eyes. Of course; I close my eyes because of the feeling I am going over Victoria Falls – as water flows liberally, only to be expertly caught in a bowl.

At last I was released. What a nice chap my dentist is – I really must invite him out to dinner soon. I did, and couldn't think of anything to say – he had conditioned me to silence over many years!

My self-confidence was shaken when, 24 hours later, reflecting on his reply, another old filling disintegrated when I inadvertently bit into a plum stone, and I had to return to have it replaced.

A dentist's chair is a good place to reflect: as he was repairing the latest mishap, I thought about my dentist's comment about his intimate knowledge of only one orifice, and was reminded how a gynaecologist friend of mine was equally dedicated to his professional work, and – you might conclude, was as exclusively preoccupied, professionally, with one particular orifice as my dentist was with his. I always thought it was rather unkind of his wife when bidding him goodbye in the morning, to wish him a 'happy day at the orifice'.

But to return to my dentist: the reason I have recounted my visit to him is that he is also a philosopher. In the old days when the drill was driven by a series of cables, he would attach a small piece of cotton wool to the cable, and ask children to watch it, so distracting their attention from the 'dreaded drill'.

On this day, he was philosophising on the topic of how long one might live for and we had a (one-sided) conversation on the subject, reminding me that Jonathan Swift had some firm ideas.

Immortality

For anybody having lingering doubts about the desirability of living a s t r e t c h e d life, I would recommend to them Swift's *A Voyage to Laputa* from *Gulliver's Travels*. In Chapter Ten, Gulliver describes how he stayed with the Luggnuggians, and met with the small group called Struldbruggs, who were immortal and could be identified by a small black spot on their foreheads. As Swift says...

> *...long life is the universal Desire and Wish of Mankind. That whoever had one foot in the Grave, was sure to hold back the other as strongly as he could. That the oldest had still Hopes of living one Day longer, and looked on Death as the greatest Evil...*

The difficulties of being immortal should be read in the context that Swift's tales were written in – the early eighteenth century, when longevity was the exception: to have reached forty, one was considered to be old. As seen through Swift's imaginative, but practical pen, the Luggnuggians laid down strict rules to contain these unwanted perpetual citizens. Swift spoke for mortals when he was asked by his hosts how he would see himself, and utilise the gift of immortality. Unhesitantly, he said he would first make himself rich, and by thrift and good monetary management would become the richest man in the Kingdom within 200 years ('Argentosis' do I hear you say? Then turn to Chapter Seven). His second ambition would be to become more learned than anybody else, and thirdly, to become more wise 'and so become the oracle of the Nation'.

Perhaps the sage thing about Swift is that he then drew up the disadvantages of immortality, namely that immortality did not confer immunity from the very serious shortcomings of getting old, 'degeneracy' as he put it. Swift concluded that – as seen through the experiences of the Struldbruggs – those doomed to immortality would behave as other mortals until they reached 30 years of age. They then would become increasingly melancholic and dejected, until they reached the age of 80 which was considered to be the 'Extremity of Living'. At this age, the Struldbruggs had:

> ...not only the Follies and Infirmities of other old Men, but many more which arose from the dreadful Prospect of never dying. They were not only opinionated, peevish, covetous, morose, vain, talkative, but incapable of Friendship and Dead to all natural affection.

He also referred to 'Envy and impotent Desires' and 'being cut off from any possibility of pleasure.' As for the sight of a funeral, they would 'repine that others had gone to the Harbour of Rest to which they themselves never can hope to aspire.' Swift surely would have been a protagonist for voluntary euthanasia. He also mentions that the more fortunate Struldbruggs were those who lost their memories ('in their dotage'), for they were no longer distressed – an unwitting reference to Alzheimer's disease.

Swift also made a cynical reference to marriage, in that, in the event of two Struldbruggs marrying, the marriage would be dissolved at the age of 80, 'for they should not have their misery doubled by the Load of a wife', and at the same age they should be declared 'dead in Law to enable their Heirs to inherit their Estate, with but a small pittance reserved for their support.'

Swift goes on to spell out some of the disadvantages of advanced old age:

> ...at Ninety they lose their teeth, hair, and taste. Consequently they eat and drink whatever they can get, without relish... forget Names of Persons, even their relatives. Similarly they cannot read, for their Memory cannot serve to carry them from the Beginning of a Sentence to the End, and after 200 years cannot conduct a conversation (other than a few words), and are therefore like foreigners in their own land.

Swift concludes that '...from what I have seen, my keen appetite for perpetuity of life is much abated, and no death could be devised which would not be preferable.'

For those diehards still determined to stay around at life's party when all others have departed, Swift offers the following guidelines for the surviving very old:

Not to marry a young woman.

Not to keep their company unless they really desire it.

Not to be peevish or morose, or suspicious.

Not to scorn present Ways, or Wits, or Fashions, or Men, or War, etc.

Not to be fond of children, or let them come near me hardly.

Nor to tell the same Story over and over to the same people.

Not to be covetous.

Not to neglect decency, or cleanliness, for fear of falling into Nastiness.

Not to be severe with young People, but give allowances for their Youthful Follies, and Weaknesses.

Not to be influenced by, or give ear to knavish tattling servants or others.

Not to be too free of advice nor trouble any but those that desire it.

To desire some good Friends to inform me which of these Resolutions I break, or neglect, and wherein; and reform accordingly.

Not to talk much, nor of myself.

Not to boast of my former beauty, or strength, or favour with Ladies etc.

Not to hearken to Flatteries,

Nor conceive I can be loved by a Young Woman.

Not to be positive or opiniative.

Not to set up for observing all these Rules for fear I should observe none.

Jonathan Swift (1667–1745)

And for the cynically inclined:

Sleep is good; death is better; but, of course, best of all would be never to have been born at all.

Heinrich Heine (1797–1856)

Self-Determination

The subject of voluntary euthanasia is discussed in a separate chapter, but nearly everyone has in an transitory moment expressed a thought about 'wishing it would all end'.

Such a thought would seem to be diametrically opposed to the spirit of this book. But is it? Not completely.

'Can't you stay, must you go?' is an old conundrum suggesting you should! Whatever the answer, I believe it is fundamental that one should retain the ultimate decision over one's own final destiny.

In contemplating this decision, i.e., to terminate as opposed to laying down a policy for extending life (by modifying one's lifestyle), one should read the voluntary euthanasia section.

The most important factor in deciding to live a little longer by avoiding those illnesses causing premature death, is that (death being inevitable) to avoid one cause of death is, by definition, to opt for another. The alternative death may be more unpleasant and more painful, less dignified, and less acceptable. The result of declining the option as one disease is avoided is that all the others remain, one or more of which will come to claim you.

Look at Figure XIII again. Regard it as a menu: 25% of those illnesses are smoking-related.

Remember that three of the commonest premature life-threatening illnesses can to a considerable extent be avoided (road traffic accidents, heart attacks, suicides). To these should be added the long list of smoking-related deaths (25% of all deaths).

Contemplate the manner of dying from these 'voluntary' deaths, i.e., quickly or with a degree of pain and suffering. They should still be avoided, though, for 'life's rich tapestry' will surely have much left to offer.

Having decided to take a chance on the alternatives awaiting your despatch, cast your eye over them and consider how you might avoid the worst should something unacceptable turn up.

DNA Genetic Testing.

(Deoxyribonucleic acid: the self-regulating material present in nearly all living organisms, chromosomes, carriers of genetic information.)

Though still at an early stage in development, DNA testing can give with some degree of accuracy an estimate of life expectancy as well as a guide on the probability of developing cancer. Already there are protests that using this would be an invasion of privacy as well as an intrusion on human rights. This latter because anybody who is found to have inherited unfavourable genes will be discriminated against should an insurance life policy quotation be sought.

It would seem difficult to separate this from a case of raising the premium for somebody who is considered a high risk because he indulges in hazardous sports or has a similar dangerous lifestyle or who may even be HIV positive. Even smokers are already faced with relatively high premiums as they represent potential claims under the policy. The converse side of this argument is that the 'good risk genes' will benefit from lower premiums when taking out life assurances.

Before the discovery of DNA, such choice was already available to anybody. It is generally accepted that the chances of a cancer developing are greatly enhanced if both an intrinsic and extrinsic factor are present (such as smoking for example). The likelihood of the intrinsic factor being present can be judged by looking through the causes of death of one's older family members. If more than 40% of one's predecessors died from cancer then the chances of oneself doing the same are raised considerably. In such circumstances those same chances are considerably reduced if one avoids carcinogenic substances, of which by far the commonest is associated with smoking.

If conclusions are beginning to be drawn about how long and in what state one is likely to live, I would invite you to compare life with the popular game of Monopoly and enjoy drawing your weekly pension every time you pass 'GO'; and if your local postmaster greets you with 'You here again?', concede it possible that what he really meant was how pleasant it was to see you, rather than it being a surprise!

High morale and a sense of humour are as essential ingredients for ongoing living as petrol and oil are for your car. As you leave the post office make a mental note that it will only be another week before your return to 'top up' again.

Still want to live a little longer? Of course you do; you're human and still healthy and life is good, so get on with living and put these morbid thoughts aside.

But do not go the other extreme and indulge in things which do not appeal to you, such as fanatical exercise (remember those unsmiling, possibly dead joggers), or unappetising diets (that steak could be just the thing your body needs), or total abstention (a regular tot of alcohol will probably extend your life as well as making it more fun); in short, partake in liberal doses of moderation.

Do avoid the proven harmful habits such as smoking, one of the few harmful habits that are legal.

Having, as I suspect you have, elected to take a chance on what lies ahead for the manner of your end, get on with living, that's what life is for; cross future bridges as they come!

If you have reached 70 (or thereabouts), begin to relax some of the rules, and make sure you enjoy everything you do; you will be unlikely to begin or recommence smoking so the biggest threat is disposed of.

Seventy onwards offer truly golden years so enjoy them; you will be throttling back from full power and starting to enjoy some of the forbidden fruit. The next twenty years could be the best of all, and set your target, including financial – not forgetting the difference between 'budget' and 'target' expectation years.

Probably the zenith is reached around the age of 90, and everything that comes thereafter should be regarded as a true golden nugget, so detailed plans are probably not required, each day to be taken as it turns up.

Above all, do not covet any desires to live for ever or even for much longer after the age of 90. Remember Swift's Struldbruggs!

Having thought all these options through, you can now give your answer to the question; I have little doubt of a resounding:

'YES'

to the question:

WHY NOT LIVE A LITTLE LONGER?

...but suggest you add – 'but not too long'.

To every thing there is a season,.
A time to be born, and a time to die.

Ecclesiastes 2:13.

Before getting on with your life, remember that:

• Only three persons in ten have made a will.

• Of these, 65% are over 65.

• 12% of those who had not made a will thought they were 'too young' and maybe unlikely to die!

Please don't forget to make your will! Happy evenings, and good living to you.

Appendix I

Author's Note: I am indebted to Professor Brian Livesley for advice regarding the content of this section.

Care Of The Dying.

> *...earth to earth;*
> *ashes to ashes;*
> *dust to dust...*

Death being inevitable, it is appropriate that this book finishes on the topic just as it began by attempting to examine the nature of the subject, with life sandwiched in between.

With regard to the title itself, (*Why Not Live A Little Longer?*) it is also considered appropriate to consign this brief discourse properly to the status of an appendix, leaving the main thrust of the question intact and with a message containing hope and optimism. This admits postponement of the event, and not rejection of the concept.

From a clinical standpoint, care of the dying, once that diagnosis has been made, must maintain a considered balance between the extremes of 'heroics', implying unwarranted persistent bodily intrusion, and abandonment of a hopeless case.

Possibly more than any other medical diagnosis and the consequences thereof, the patient has a full part to play, including some determination of the timing of death. It should be regarded as natural an event as childbirth, although the two are at the extremes of life. In both cases assistance is more importance than participation.

It is a time when the hospice comes into its own, with a very special role.

500,000 deaths occur every year in the United Kingdom, of which half are aged over 74, and 20% over 84. It is significant that no one dies of 'old age', but a medical diagnosis is made in each case for statistical purposes. Thus the diagnosis and treatment of the dying has become more difficult due to temptations of the high scientific content of both diagnostic techniques and treatments now available in modern medical practice.

> *Whilst we must adhere to medicine's traditional role of life prolongation, we now have to decide in each case when this becomes an appropriate goal. Perhaps we should ask ourselves: 'What would I wish if the patient were my own mother?', or, even more pertinently: 'What if I were the patient'?*

> (Williamson, 1981)

It is also easy to fall into the trap of prescribing medicines on medicines, i.e., prescribing a further medicine without ensuring that the previous medicine has been stopped, the medicines sometimes having diametrically opposite effects, as if one were driving a car with the brakes on. The result leads to mental confusion, thus complicating the diagnosis. I recall being called in to see an old lady who was very confused and unable to recognise her daughter, and, for that matter, her daughter was unable to recognise the mother she had known. For all the world a straightforward case of dementia, until I asked to see her medicines, which I removed, saying I would see her again in a couple of days time. When I returned, the entire scene had changed and a normal elderly lady greeted me with, "How nice of you to call; we haven't met before, have we?"

To which I could only say, "Well, not really, but how nice to see you looking so well!"

When a firm diagnosis of 'dying' has been made, the most important general treatment is 'Tender Loving Care' (TLC). In the terminal stages, a form of intensive care is required in addition, rather than abandonment, if the patient is to be assisted to a gentle end. At this time it is obligatory to assess the patient's final wishes, as well as including spiritual guidance if this is required. Above all, nothing should be enforced. If the patient does not require food then give no food. Even fluids should be administered sparingly if there is evidence of fluid in the lungs causing distress.

The 'not allowed to die' syndrome should be avoided, and unnecessary resuscitation avoided.

Pain Control

Nobody should or need suffer pain, and this abhorrent suffering must be avoided. Pain control care is a specialised art. If ill-judged it can lead to mental confusion followed by increased administration of drugs, in turn exacerbating the mental confusion.

The patient may slip into a drug-induced twilight sleep possibly accompanied by unpleasant dreams. These may lead to terror hallucinations. Should this occur, a high degree of nursing skill is called for to reassure and help the patient to retain a tenuous link with reality.

Hospice

Caring for the dying is a very specialised form of nursing care sometimes requiring extended supervision over a long time. The hospice movement was pioneered in the United Kingdom.

In the cases of chronically but terminally ill patients, the sufferer is encouraged to spend a short period in the hospice before finally taking up permanent residence. This serves two purposes. It enables the patient to become accustomed to the surroundings prior to eventual admission as well as the staff of the hospice getting to know the personality of their new charge.

It also gives oft-needed respite to the relations of the terminally ill patient. "It's like going to an hotel," said one patient of mine, "and they make you feel so welcome."

Relatives

The final days, be they spent in a hospice or hospital, are most important, both for the patient as well as for close relatives who have a very clear role to play if dying is not to be a lonely time. Their role is both complementary and supplementary to nursing care. They provide social care, and can give comfort and reassurance to those in their final days and hours. They act much as a nautical pilot does before handing over to the captain of a vessel for the next stage of the journey.

At appropriate moments, if circumstances permit they should be encouraged to stay in the hospital and so be immediately at hand.

Exitus

The question of living wills or advance declarations has been covered elsewhere, but this is the time when their existence, made long before their value becomes apparent, can come into its own and be of assistance to those caring for the patient. Such a declaration made after a terminal illness becomes known may well leave a suspicion of doubt as to the real wishes of the patient.

The Demise

The moment of death does not put paid to what has to be done. Now is the time to turn attention to the survivors. They will in all probability require comfort and advice. The late patient's general practitioner will need to be informed, the death certificate issued, and a degree of comfort will not come amiss if the start of grieving is not to be another wholly trying time. The relatives may well want to pose questions and also they might have some guilt feelings as to whether they might have done more, and general bewilderment could gain hold.

Relatives, for the sake of a few moments' considerate attention on the part of nurses, can be given a real helping hand on the road back to normality. They may well want to ask questions, and also they may have some guilt feelings.

To return to the question posed in the book title, and to which I hope you can answer in the affirmative, please remember that eventually your turn will come also, but hopefully not for a little while longer.

Appendix II
The Hippocratic Oath

The origin of this declaration is usually attributed to the Greek physician Hippocrates, who lived on the Greek island of Kos some four centuries before the birth of Christ.

It was a remarkable document which has stood the test of time in its original form, but it had fallen into disuse for newly qualifying doctors and a revised, up-to-date version was issued by the World Medical Association in 1983, as follows:

> *I solemnly pledge myself to consecrate my life to the service of humanity.*
>
> *I will give to my teachers the respect and gratitude which is their due.*
>
> *I will practise my profession with conscience and dignity. The health of my patient will be my first consideration.*
>
> *I will respect the secrets which are confided in me, even after the patient has died.*
>
> *I will maintain by all the means in my power, the honour and noble traditions of the medical profession.*
>
> *My colleagues will all be my brothers.*
>
> *I will not permit considerations of religion, nationality, race, party politics, or social standing to intervene between my duty and my patients.*
>
> *I will maintain the utmost respect for human life from its beginning even under threat and I will not use my medical knowledge contrary to the laws of humanity.*
>
> *I make these promises solemnly, freely, and upon my honour.*

The British Medical Association has drawn up a revised version of the Hippocratic Oath for consideration by the World Medical Association in 1998. Ominously, on confidentiality it states only:

> ...*that doctors will* do their best to maintain confidentiality: *"If there are* overriding reasons *which prevent me keeping a patient's confidentiality, I will explain them."*

It goes on to state that:

> ...*the prolongation of human life is not the only aim of health care.*

The first of these two statements would appear to be yet another instance of eroding the 'human private area' (see Chapter Six).

Appendix III
Letter To The Editor

Sir,

Politicians, and certain others who should know better, often find it convenient to place anyone living beyond the age of 70 into a special 'unrepairable' category. But they should take note of the future voting power of such categories.

In 1951 there were 300 centenarians, in 2011 there will be in excess of 25,000. In 1961 there were 300,000 people over 85, in 2012 there will be 1.3 million over 85. The number of pensioners will exceed 16 million by 2031 – more than double the number in 1961.

It is disheartening for those people who do not feel or consider themselves 'old' to be bombarded with newspaper articles referring to 'caring for the elderly' and the like. It would be more constructive to concentrate instead on how much the 'elderly' might contribute. A considerable number of those over 75 are physically able, mentally alert and independent. We should recognise the contribution that they could make – not just to society, but to the Gross National Product.

The senior generations must resist the temptation of being talked into 'being old' prematurely – that is a sure recipe for curtailing life itself.

My own speciality is gerontology, the study of the ageing process, and not to be confused with geriatrics, which deals with the health and care of old people. In collecting material for a forthcoming book, Why Not

Live a Little Longer?, *I have case records of over 10,000 patients, mostly from the upper age groups. One particularly worthy of mention concerns an ex-pilot, who regained his licence at the age of 72 after an absence from flying of over 30 years. His only disappointment was that it took him nearly five hours to go solo, compared with four hours in 1946.*

I have noted that a large proportion of my cases are getting a lot of fun out of life. I fully intend to emulate them and would like to suggest the following age definitions as a practical guide. Middle-aged: 45-65, elderly: 65-85, and old: over 85. The term 'geriatric' should be reserved for describing a medical condition, not chronological age.

As a maxim, I would quote that eminent physician Denis Burkitt:

Attitudes are more important than abilities.
Motives are more important than methods.
Character is important than cleverness.
Perseverance is more important than power.
And the heart takes precedence over the head.

Dr Herbert Ellis
High Hurstwood, Sussex